Positive Options for Living with COPD

Titles in the Positive Options for Health Series

Positive Options
for
Living with COPD

**Self-Help and Treatment for
Chronic Obstructive Pulmonary Disease**

Teri Allen, RRT

Hunter House
PUBLISHERS

Hunter House Inc., Publishers
PO Box 2914
Alameda CA 94501-0914

All figures with the exception of
Figures 6.1, 7.1, and 9.1 are from LifeARTCollection
© 1980–2001 by Lippincott Williams & Wilkins, Baltimore, MD.

Library of Congress Cataloging-in-Publication Data
Allen, Teri Ann.
Positive options for living with COPD : self-help and treatment for chronic obstructive pulmonary disease / by Teri Allen. — 1st ed.
p. cm. — (Positive options for health)
Includes bibliographical references and index.
ISBN 978-0-89793-553-1 (pbk.)
1. Lungs—Diseases, Obstructive—Popular works. I. Title.
RC776.O3A45 2010
616.2'4—dc22   2010002068

Project Credits
Cover Design: Stefanie Gold   Publicity Coordinator: Sean Harvey
Book Production: John McKercher   Rights Coordinator: Candace Groskreutz
Copy Editor: Mary Miller   Order Fulfillment: Washul Lakdhon
Proofreader: John David Marion   Administrator: Theresa Nelson
Indexer: Nancy D. Peterson   Computer Support: Peter Eichelberger
Editor: Alexandra Mummery   Senior Marketing Associate: Reina Santana
Customer Service Manager: Christina Sverdrup
Publisher: Kiran S. Rana

Printed and bound by Sheridan Books, Ann Arbor, Michigan
Manufactured in the United States of America

9 8 7 6 5 4 3 2 1   First Edition   10 11 12 13 14

DEDICATION

● ● ●

This book is dedicated to all of the wonderful patients
that I have worked with over the years who have risen
above their lung disease to live happy, fulfilled lives.

Your bravery and courage are an inspiration to all of those
who suffer from chronic obstructive pulmonary disease.

Ordering

Trade bookstores in the U.S. and Canada please contact:

Publishers Group West
1700 Fourth Street, Berkeley CA 94710
Phone: (800) 788-3123   Fax: (800) 351-5073

Hunter House books are available at bulk discounts for textbook
course adoptions; to qualifying community, health-care, and government
organizations; and for special promotions and fund-raising.
For details please contact:

Special Sales Department
Hunter House Inc., PO Box 2914, Alameda CA 94501-0914
Phone: (510) 865-5282   Fax: (510) 865-4295
E-mail: ordering@hunterhouse.com

Individuals can order our books from most bookstores, by calling
(800) 266-5592, or from our website at **www.hunterhouse.com**

Contents

● ● ●

Preface: Reclaim Your Life

● ● ●

This life is yours. You were given a body in which to live. This body will have limitations. All bodies do, and there is not one human being on this earth who is perfect. Some limitations are physical. Others are mental. The key to optimal living is to work with your limitations rather than against them.

Imagine swimming in the ocean. Which is easier—fighting against each wave as it crashes toward you or using the momentum of the waves to push you ashore until your feet are on solid ground?

Having limitations can leave us with a sense of loneliness, frustration, anger, or depression. These reactions are perfectly normal. However, regaining a sense of control over your limitations is the key to managing your chronic obstructive pulmonary disease (COPD).

How do we regain a sense of control when it feels as if our limitations control us? We do so by making the choice to live. We do so by making the commitment to take care of ourselves. We do so by setting goals, sticking to them, and monitoring our progress. We do so by building support systems to help us get through times when we are feeling down, discouraged, or frustrated. We do so by asking for help, when we need it. And finally, we do so by letting go of past beliefs and building new ones that allow us to overcome our limitations and get on with living.

Successful management of COPD requires commitment. Before you read further, you must ask yourself an important question: "Am I committed to feeling better?" You *can* and *will* be able to make a significant difference in the quality of your life if you make the commitment to take an active role in managing your disease.

The diagnosis of COPD can be devastating. Just as in other areas of our life, when we are faced with making significant changes in our lifestyle, there are conflicting emotions. This is normal. Each person's feelings about the diagnosis are different and depend on a variety of factors. Just know this: Having COPD is not a death sentence. With proper disease management, you can expect to live a full and happy life.

There is no magic pill or quick fix for COPD. However, there are many things you can do to have more energy, less-frequent shortness of breath, and an overall better quality of life.

Quality of life is difficult to define. Simply put, it means living your life to the fullest extent possible. It is enjoying your life, despite your degree of breathlessness or your use of home oxygen. You do have physical limitations. But doesn't everybody? Some of us are short, others are tall, some are heavy, some are frail—but we manage to work around these limitations in all situations and live life well. You can learn to work with your problems rather than fighting against them.

Take a moment to think about the things you enjoyed doing before the symptoms of COPD began affecting your life. Perhaps you feel you cannot garden or golf anymore because you are too short of breath or embarrassed by your coughing. Perhaps your problem is as simple as being unable to shower or apply makeup without breathlessness. Find a piece of paper and write down three things you would like to be able to do well again, without experiencing overwhelming episodes of breathlessness.

These three things are important to you. There may be obstacles to overcome, but if your goals are realistic and you are committed to feeling better, there is no reason you cannot do these things again.

Goals are an important aspect of everyone's life. Without goals, we are unable to track our progress along life's journey. In order to achieve our goals, we need certain tools to help us along the way, and this book will help you achieve your personal goal of improving your quality of life by doing the following:

- providing you with information about your disease so that you can understand *why* you feel the way you do

- helping you address the psychological and emotional issues that go along with having COPD and which can be stumbling blocks in the pathway to feeling better

- helping you organize your personal health information so that you can get the most help from your health-care providers
- showing you how to learn to identify those things that make your breathing worse
- allowing you to recognize the warning signs of worsening symptoms and encouraging the creation of an action plan
- teaching you techniques that will make breathing easier

Your challenge is no different from that of an athlete. An athlete must first decide on a goal. Perhaps the goal is winning a 10K or a marathon. The athlete must then build his team of experts to help him achieve his goals. He gathers information about how to best train his body and learns skills that will make him a winner. He practices what he learns every day, with his team by his side cheering him on. With commitment and hard work, he will win. Maybe he will not win the first race, and maybe not the second, but with time and practice he will become a winner. And so will you!

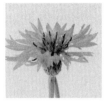

CHAPTER 1

Understanding the Respiratory System

The first step toward effective disease management is to become familiar with the body parts involved. Learning about the respiratory system will make it easier for you to understand the terminology used by your health-care providers. This will enable you to better understand your disease, as well as to learn why your health-care provider prescribes different treatments and how mismanagement can affect other body systems, which may further complicate the disease process.

The Respiratory System

The respiratory system is both sophisticated and delicate. It supplies your body with the oxygen it needs to survive. Without the oxygen you take in with every breath, you would die within minutes.

Every cell in your body needs oxygen to survive. Oxygen allows the cells to extract energy from the food you eat. Without oxygen the body has no energy, and as a result—no life.

About 20 percent of the air you breathe is oxygen. The rest is comprised of nitrogen and trace gases. When the oxygen supply reaches your cells, it combines with food to produce energy. The waste products from this reaction are water and carbon dioxide. Carbon dioxide is toxic to the body. The respiratory system rids the body of carbon dioxide by exhalation.

In simple terms: When you inhale, you take in oxygen, which is carried to the cells and creates energy for your body (see Figure 1.1).When you exhale, carbon dioxide is eliminated from the body, preventing toxic results. This process is called *gas exchange*, or *oxygen transport.*

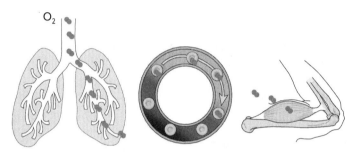

FIGURE 1.1: *The oxygen transport system. Oxygen is taken in through the lungs, passes through the capillary system, and travels on to the skeletal muscles.*

The Upper Airway

The upper airway consists of the nose and the mouth (see Figure 1.2). The nose functions to warm, filter, and humidify the air you breathe. Inside the nose are many tiny hairs that filter out dust, smoke, and other foreign particles that you may inhale. The nose is lined with *mucus* to help trap these particles. When you sneeze or blow your nose, these particles are expelled.

In addition, the warm, moist surface of the inside of the nasal cavity humidifies and warms the air that you breathe before it reaches your lower airways.

The Lower Airway

After air passes through your nose or mouth, it continues on through the windpipe (*trachea*). The trachea is lined with *cartilage*, making the passageway very strong and rigid.

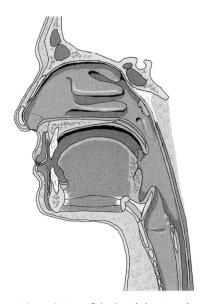

FIGURE 1.2: *A lateral view of the head showing the anatomy associated with the upper respiratory system.*

The trachea divides into two branches, like a tree (Figure 1.3). The branches are called the right and left *bronchi*. Like the nasal cavity, they are lined with mucus and hairlike structures called *cilia*, which further protect your lungs from foreign particles. Coughing usually brings up the mucus that has collected for elimination.

The bronchial tubes continue to branch into smaller and smaller tubes (airways). Bands of muscle wrap around these smaller tubes. Air travels through these branches until it reaches the smallest airways, which are called bronchioles.

The bronchioles end in saclike structures, which are called *alveoli*

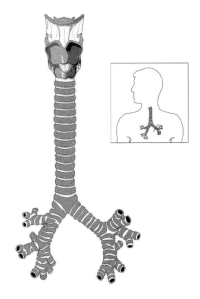

FIGURE 1.3: *The trachea and bronchi*

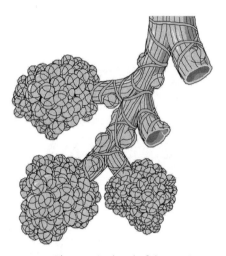

FIGURE 1.4: *The terminal end of the respiratory tract showing bronchioles and alveoli.*

(see Figure 1.4). This is where the oxygen and carbon dioxide exchange occurs. Healthy lungs usually have 300 million alveoli (air sacs), which are similar to balloons.

The blood vessels that surround the alveoli absorb oxygen into the bloodstream. They also allow carbon dioxide to be removed from the blood. Carbon dioxide enters the alveoli and is exhaled (see Figure 1.4).

Blood travels through these tiny blood vessels into larger vessels that eventually empty into the left side of the heart. This oxygen-rich blood is then carried to every cell of the body.

When the blood returns to the right side of the heart, it is full of carbon dioxide that needs to be eliminated. The blood is pumped from the right side of the heart through the lungs and the exchange of oxygen and carbon dioxide occurs (see Figure 1.5).

How Breathing Works

With healthy lungs, little work goes into the act of breathing. The huge band of muscle below the rib cage, called the *diaphragm*, contracts and pulls air into the lungs. As the diaphragm relaxes, air is exhaled with no effort at all.

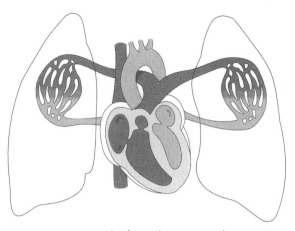

FIGURE 1.5: *A schematic representation of pulmonary circulation.*

How Breathing Is Controlled

The brain is the control center for breathing. The body sends signals to the brain when carbon dioxide levels increase above normal levels. The brain tells the body to breathe faster and/or deeper to get rid of the excess carbon dioxide. This is most noticeable during exercise. As the muscles use more oxygen for energy, there is more carbon dioxide waste to be removed. The brain senses this and tells the body to breathe harder and faster.

How the Heart and Lungs Work Together

The heart and lungs work together to keep the body supplied with oxygen. When the heart and lungs are working together properly, our body gets the oxygen it needs and we are healthy. But if one of them becomes diseased or damaged, the other has to work harder to compensate and keep the body in balance.

Two things happen when the lungs are damaged:

1. Lack of oxygen makes the heart pump harder and faster in an effort to keep the oxygen levels normal. At first, the heart muscle is strong and can keep up with the work. But the

heart is not made to work this hard and this fast for long periods of time. Eventually, the heart becomes tired and weak.

2. Additionally, in response to *hypoxia* (low blood-oxygen levels), the tiny blood vessels in the lungs constrict (become smaller). This constriction creates resistance to blood flow. Back flow creates strain on the heart muscle and weakens it. This can lead to right-sided heart failure (*cor pulmonale*). Some people with COPD have this complication as well.

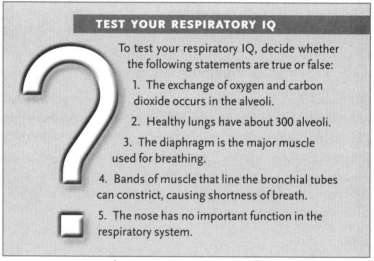

TEST YOUR RESPIRATORY IQ

To test your respiratory IQ, decide whether the following statements are true or false:

1. The exchange of oxygen and carbon dioxide occurs in the alveoli.

2. Healthy lungs have about 300 alveoli.

3. The diaphragm is the major muscle used for breathing.

4. Bands of muscle that line the bronchial tubes can constrict, causing shortness of breath.

5. The nose has no important function in the respiratory system.

(Answers: 1:T 2:F 3:T 4:T 5:F)

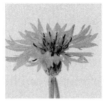

CHAPTER 2

What Is COPD?

You are probably reading this book because you or someone you love has breathing problems. You may have been given a diagnosis of *emphysema, chronic bronchitis,* or *chronic asthma.* All of these conditions have one thing in common—*airway obstruction.* People with COPD either have trouble getting air into or out of their lungs. This can cause a wide range of symptoms, but they are all related to airway obstruction.

COPD is suspected when certain symptoms are present, especially when combined with a history of smoking and/or an exposure to particles such as dust, chemicals, or fumes while on the job.

People exposed to indoor air pollution, such as heating supplied by a woodstove, or to high levels of outdoor industrial air pollution are also at risk for developing COPD, especially if combined with a history of smoking.

Symptoms and tolerance to COPD vary from person to person. However, most people share some common symptoms, including:

- a cough that is chronic and productive of *sputum*
- repeated episodes of acute bronchitis
- shortness of breath that becomes worse over time, is present every day, and becomes worse with exercise or during respiratory infections

A diagnosis of COPD must be confirmed through *spirometry* testing, which is described in more detail in Chapter 3. An accurate diagnosis is important so that the most effective treatment can be prescribed. COPD is a combination of three disorders—chronic bronchitis, emphysema, and chronic (or bronchial) asthma—all of which disturb the airflow through the respiratory system.

Chronic Bronchitis

Chronic bronchitis is identified when an individual has a productive cough for three months or more over a two-year period. It is different from acute bronchitis because chronic bronchitis does not go away. It usually develops due to smoking, occupational exposure to irritants, or frequent childhood respiratory infections.

Chronic irritation of the bronchi creates *inflammation* of the bronchial lining. This inflammation narrows the airways (see Figure 2.1). It also leads to excess mucus production, resulting in a "smoker's cough."

The lungs produce excess mucus as a defense against inhaled irritants. Normally, the excess mucus would trap small particles be-

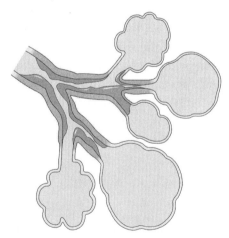

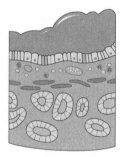

cross-section of epithelium where bronchitis is taking place

sagittal section of respiratory bronchiole and alveoli suffering from chronic bronchitis

FIGURE 2.1: *Chronic bronchitis*

fore they enter the lungs and would then be coughed out. Chronic irritation and inflammation result in an increase in mucus production cells as the body tries harder and harder to defend the lungs. This excess mucus becomes difficult to cough up and becomes trapped in the narrow, inflamed airways, thus leading to obstruction.

Trapped mucus is the perfect breeding ground for bacteria, and this puts you at risk for lung infections such as *pneumonia* (see Figure 2.2).

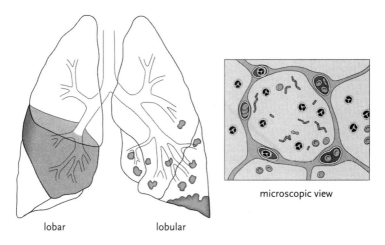

lobar   lobular

FIGURE 2.2: *Lungs showing two types of pneumonia (left) lobar and (right) lobular. Microscopic view shows bacteria responsible for fluid build-up.*

People with chronic bronchitis may experience shortness of breath. The degree of breathlessness depends upon the amount of airway congestion and irritation. Periods of flare-up (*exacerbation*) usually follow an upper respiratory infection and symptoms may become more noticeable at this time.

Emphysema

While chronic bronchitis mainly involves the bronchial tree, emphysema involves the lower airways, especially the bronchioles and the alveoli. Constant exposure to irritants causes the bronchioles to lose their elasticity, which causes them to narrow and collapse. The

alveoli are damaged as well, which stretches out and destroys the
delicate air sacs (see Figure 2.3).

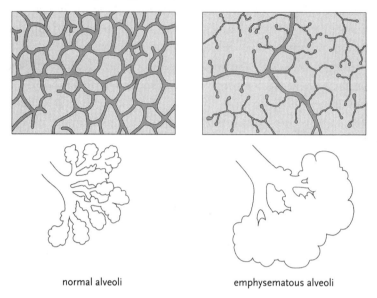

normal alveoli   emphysematous alveoli

FIGURE 2.3: *Emphysema*

Our body's defense system can cause a lot of the damage seen
with emphysema. In healthy lungs, an enzyme is released to prevent
lung damage from invaders such as bacteria. This enzyme eats bacteria. But if too much enzyme is released in a defensive reaction, the
enzyme will also eat the lung tissue and leave holes.

In healthy lungs, chemicals are released to block the effects of
damage from this bacteria-eating enzyme. Cigarette smoking dis-
rupts the body's normal defense system and results in overproduc-
tion of the enzyme. The enzyme runs wild and eats lung tissue, resulting in a type of "Swiss cheese" effect in the lungs.

In addition to smoking, there is a rare genetic cause for emphysema. The enzyme that blocks the effect is lacking at birth and emphysema develops in the same way as it does for those who smoke.
This type of emphysema is called alpha$_1$-antitrypsin disorder.

Either way, damage and destruction of lung tissue makes it difficult for the body to absorb oxygen or to eliminate carbon dioxide.

Obstruction of the airways also occurs. Once the bronchioles lose their elasticity, or structure, they tend to collapse, leaving air trapped in the alveoli. This allows carbon dioxide to build up.

Much of the breathlessness experienced by people with emphysema is caused by this "air trapping," which causes the lungs to *hyperinflate*. The lungs push the diaphragm flat as they fill with trapped air. With no room to contract, the diaphragm cannot do much to help with breathing. *Accessory muscles* located in the neck, shoulders, and upper back take over this work. With all this extra effort to breathe, no wonder people with emphysema are tired!

Alpha₁-Antitrypsin Disorder

Alpha$_1$-antitrypsin disorder is a genetic condition that causes emphysema-like changes in the lungs. It is not caused by smoking or exposure to damaging particles in the air but by a deficiency in alpha$_1$-antitrypsin. This enzyme is produced in the liver and is designed to protect the lungs from damage caused by infection or inhaled irritants, as well as to heal lung tissue.

A deficiency in this important enzyme may result in destruction of alveoli at an early age. It may also cause liver cirrhosis due to the enzyme accumulating abnormally in the liver. It is important to be tested for this genetic condition, especially if there is a family of the disease or if COPD is diagnosed at an early age.

Treatment for this disease includes weekly intravenous therapy with a solution that replaces the lacking enzyme. It can be given at the hospital on an outpatient basis, in a clinic, or in the home. Talk with your health-care provider to determine the best option for you.

Bronchial or Chronic Asthma

Unlike chronic bronchitis or emphysema, smoking does not typically cause chronic asthma. *Allergens* or irritants usually cause it. Sensitivity to these allergens is often called *reactive airway disease*. Reactive airways are a common component of COPD.

Pure asthma is treated with medications called *bronchodilators* and/or steroids. The changes that occur in the lungs are reversible.

When reactive airways are a part of COPD, the changes in the lungs cannot be reversed as easily. However, the symptoms *can* be controlled.

In reactive airway disease, the lining of the airways becomes inflamed and swollen. The bands of muscle lining the bronchi constrict in reaction to an inhaled irritant. This "tightening" of the muscles leads to obstruction of airflow (see Figure 2.4).

There are many types of allergens that cause chronic asthma. Some common allergens are:

- pollen
- dust
- animal hair and dander
- strong odors
- mold
- fungus
- cold air

Common symptoms of reactive airway disease are:

- shortness of breath
- wheezing
- chest tightness
- cough

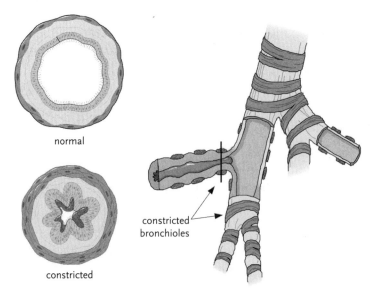

normal

constricted

constricted bronchioles

FIGURE 2.4: *Bronchial or chronic asthma*

Do I Really Have COPD?

If you suspect that you have COPD, it is vital to seek appropriate medical care. See your health-care provider if you have any of the following risk factors or symptoms of COPD:

- You are over age forty-five and have a history of smoking, occupational exposure to irritants, or frequent childhood respiratory infections.
- You have a chronic cough with little or no mucus production.
- You have a chronic cough that produces large amounts of mucus.
- You become breathless with or without exertion.
- You have difficulty exhaling fully.
- You are tired every day.
- You have experienced unexplained weight loss.

As you have just learned, COPD is an equal opportunity disease. Mary Sue was shocked when her doctor told her she had chronic obstructive pulmonary disease: "I couldn't believe it. I'd never smoked a day in my life. But he told me it was probably from all my years of waitressing down at the Lodge. It was secondhand smoke that did me in."

CHAPTER 3

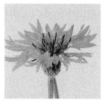

Diagnosing COPD

An early diagnosis of COPD is the cornerstone to restoring good health. Once the condition is identified, measures can be taken to reduce or reverse damage to the lungs. The progressive nature of COPD cannot be stopped or minimized until the disease is identified and properly treated.

The most important thing you can do if you have COPD is develop a good relationship with your health-care provider. Be sure to provide him or her with a complete and accurate health history in order to receive care tailored to your individual health needs.

The Physical Exam

Although a diagnosis of COPD cannot be made by a physical exam alone, your health-care provider will look for things that are common in people with chronic lung disease, such as the following:

A wider than normal chest: This is also called "barrel chest" and may indicate air trapping.

Prominent neck muscles: This may indicate that you are using accessory muscles to breathe, rather than using your diaphragm.

Weight gain or loss: Using extra energy to breathe often causes weight

---

COMMON QUESTIONS

Q: *I have been told that I am a CO_2 retainer. What does this mean?*

A: When the small bronchial tubes become floppy, inflamed, or constricted, stale air becomes trapped in the alveoli. This air contains carbon dioxide that would normally be exhaled and eliminated. Over time, the carbon dioxide levels in your blood also become elevated, causing changes in the acid/base balance of your body. These changes may also affect how your brain senses when to direct breathing. Those with CO_2 retention may actually stop breathing when oxygen saturation levels become higher than 94 percent. Although this scenario is rare, it highlights the importance of using home oxygen exactly as your health-care provider has prescribed.

Q: *What causes shortness of breath? Does shortness of breath mean I need extra oxygen?*

A: Most people think that low oxygen levels cause shortness of breath, but studies have shown that many people with hypoxia do not experience any shortness of breath at all until it becomes severe. Several factors can contribute to the feeling of shortness of breath. These include:

- increased work of breathing either due to weakened respiratory muscles or loss of elasticity in the lungs, which causes resistance
- chemical receptors in the brain that sense increased carbon dioxide levels
- increased cardiac workload due to a weakened, damaged, or enlarged heart muscle

---

loss. Weight gain may occur due to edema caused by the extra work placed on your heart.

The color of your lips, nail beds, or skin: A bluish tinge to any of these areas may indicate a low blood oxygen level.

Breathing pattern: Breathing may be rapid or labored, indicating shortness of breath or increased work of breathing.

Swollen ankles: Edema (water buildup in the tissues) may cause the ankles to swell.

Your health-care provider will listen to your lungs with a stethoscope. He or she is listening for any or all of the following:

Wheezing: This may indicate constriction or obstruction of your airways. It sounds like a whistle.

Rhonchi: This may indicate obstruction or excess mucus. This is something like a wheeze, only the sound produced is deeper and more like a rumble.

Crackles: This may indicate air trapping. This sounds like Velcro strips being pulled apart. The popping sound is caused by the collapsed alveoli inflating during a deep breath.

Other vital signs that may be recorded include the following:

Blood pressure: Hypertension (increased blood pressure) may be associated with COPD.

Pulse: A rapid heart rate may be present with COPD.

Oximetry: This measures the amount of oxygen circulating through your bloodstream. Many people with COPD have low blood oxygen levels.

Your health-care provider might also conduct additional tests such as the following:

Alpha$_1$-antitrypsin deficiency screening: This test is used to rule out this genetic disorder as a cause of your COPD.

Electrocardiogram (EKG): This is performed to rule out heart disease as the cause of your shortness of breath.

Arterial blood gases (ABGs): Blood is removed with a needle from the artery in your wrist or arm. The test measures the oxygen level in your blood and how well your lungs are able to remove carbon dioxide.

Chest X ray (CXR): While the CXR is often normal in the early stages of COPD, in cases of more advanced disease it may show flattening of the diaphragm, indicating air trapping.

Lung Function Testing

Everyone with a diagnosis of COPD should have lung function testing. According to Thomas Petty, MD, a leading expert in the diagnosis and treatment of COPD, "Measurement of FEV_1 and FVC is the only simple and easy method of spotting early COPD." Early diagnosis and treatment has been proven to slow or stop the progression of the disease. The National Lung Health Institute (NLHI) has recommended that everyone over age forty-five with a smoking history be screened for COPD with spirometry. Spirometry measures the amount of air exhaled, or forced, out of your lungs. This test may be performed in your health-care provider's office or in the outpatient department of your local hospital.

A respiratory therapist will administer the test. It is very simple, but the test requires your full effort to obtain the most accurate result. Be sure to ask your health-care provider if you should take your respiratory medications on the day of the test.

You will be given a mouthpiece to blow into that is attached by a tube to a machine. The machine measures airflow. You will be given a pair of nose clips to prevent air from leaving through your nose during the test. The respiratory therapist will have you put on the nose clips and take in as deep a breath as possible. You will then place the mouthpiece in your mouth and make a tight seal with your lips. The respiratory therapist will then tell you to blow all the air out of your lungs as hard and fast as you can. It is important to keep blowing as long and as hard as you can until it feels like there is absolutely no air left in your lungs. You may need to do this several times to obtain the most accurate reading.

The machine measures your airflow and compares it to normal readings based on age, gender, and ethnic background. Three numbers will be recorded. You should know these numbers and keep a record of them. These are the following:

- FEV_1: Measures the amount of air you blow out of your lungs in one second. It is a good indicator of true lung age as well as early small airway damage.

- FVC: Measures the total amount of air blown out. Numbers lower than normal may indicate air trapping.
- FEV_1/FVC: This is a ratio of the above. It is an excellent indicator of small airway health and function.

FEV_1 is used to identify COPD. If your FEV_1 is 70 percent of normal, your COPD is considered mild. The range of 50 to 69 percent of normal indicates moderate lung damage. Less than 50 percent indicates severe COPD.

If your FEV_1/FVC is low but your FEV_1 and FVC are within normal range, this score may indicate the beginning stages of COPD. Once again, early identification and treatment of COPD is critical. COPD progresses slowly over a thirty- to forty-year time span, so the earlier COPD is caught the better.

Sometimes your spirometry will include pre- and postbronchodilator testing. After your first test, you will be given an inhaled bronchodilator. You will then blow into the tube again. This test is used to identify reactive airways that may respond to medication. If your airflow improves after receiving the inhaled medication, your health-care provider may add a bronchodilator to your medication regime.

Take a moment to write down your numbers. If you do not know them, ask your health-care provider to provide them during your next visit.

CHAPTER 4

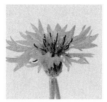

Medications:
What They Are
and How to Use Them

With so many medications now available to treat COPD, it is easy to become confused about how and when to take them. With dwindling insurance reimbursement, many health-care practitioners simply do not have the time to thoroughly review the medications they prescribe. Understanding your medication is key to managing your symptoms effectively and feeling better. It is equally important to take your medication exactly as your health-care provider has prescribed. Many times people start to feel better and stop using their medication. They do not realize that the medication is responsible for reducing or eliminating their symptoms.

The medication prescribed for COPD is not a cure. It is a part of your treatment plan for optimal health. The only way to maintain optimal health is to continue taking your medication as recommended. Changes in dose or frequency should be discussed with your health-care provider. Some medications take from several days to several months to begin working. If you stop taking your medication you may feel fine at first, but there may be a gradual decline in your overall lung health.

Bronchodilators

Bronchodilators are often prescribed for those with COPD. They are typically inhaled and help relax the constricted muscles in the airways that cause breathing difficulty. They may also help to clear mucus from the lungs by stimulating the small hairlike structures (cilia) that line the upper airways to move secretions into the upper airways where they are easier to cough out.

There are three classes of bronchodilators. Each work on different areas of the lungs to open up the airways. These include *beta-agonists*, *anticholinergics*, and *mast cell inhibitors*.

Beta-Agonists (B_2-Adrenergics)

Beta-agonists bind to receptors on the smooth muscle of the bronchial tubes, causing the muscles to relax. When used regularly, they may decrease shortness of breath, improve lung function, and prevent exacerbations of COPD.

There are two types of beta-agonists. Fast-acting beta-agonists work quickly to open your airways. They work within minutes and are effective from four to six hours.

Long-acting beta-agonists do not work as quickly but their effects last for many hours. Taken consistently, they may improve lung function, decrease shortness of breath, and make it possible for you to use your fast-acting beta-agonists less often.

■ Fast-Acting Bronchodilators

Fast-acting bronchodilators work quickly to open your airways and are often called "rescue medications." Sometimes they are combined with other types of bronchodilators to provide better relief of symptoms. Examples of fast-acting bronchodilators are:

- albuterol sulfate (Proventil, Ventolin, ProAir)
- levalbuterol (Xopenex)

Side effects include increased heart rate, shakiness, nausea, and nervousness. These effects can be minimized by rinsing your mouth with water after taking the medication.

▓ Long-Acting Bronchodilators

Long-acting beta-agonists also relax and open your airways. However, they should not be taken for immediate relief because they take effect more slowly and last longer than the fast-acting type. These are often called "maintenance" medications. Examples of long-acting bronchodilators are:

- salmeterol (Serevent)
- formoterol (Foradil)

Do not take these medications for quick relief. Instead, take your fast-acting bronchodilator. Do not take these medications more often than prescribed.

Side effects are similar to those of short-acting bronchodilators and include increased heart rate, nausea, dry mouth, and shakiness. Rinse your mouth with water after taking a treatment if these side effects are affecting you.

Anticholinergics

This type of bronchodilator blocks certain receptor sites on the smooth muscle of the bronchial tubes to prevent *bronchospasm*. They help improve smooth muscle tone, which may facilitate expiratory flow, decrease *hyperinflation*, and increase exercise tolerance. They may be combined with either long- or fast-acting beta-agonists because they work together for better effect, especially during an exacerbation of your COPD. Examples of anticholinergic bronchodilators include:

- ipratropium bromide (Atrovent): fast acting and long acting; effects last approximately six hours
- tiotropium bromide (Spiriva): long acting; effects last approximately twenty-four hours

The side effects of anticholinergics include dry mouth, blurred vision, glaucoma, and dry cough.

Mast Cell Inhibitors

Mast cells are released during the inflammatory process. Inhibiting the release of these cells can help reduce inflammation and reactions in the airways. Mast cell inhibitors must be taken exactly as prescribed to experience maximum effect. They are not to be considered "fast acting" and should not be taken in an emergency. Examples of mast cell inhibitors are:

- cromolyn sodium (Intal)
- nedocromil sodium (Tilade)

The side effects of mast cell inhibitors include headache, nausea, and nasal congestion.

Methylxanthines

Once used widely for treating those with COPD, this type of bronchodilator is no longer considered a first-line drug due to the potential for serious cardiac side effects. Taken orally, methylxanthines work to relax the smooth muscle in the airways, stimulate the centers of the brain that control breathing, and increase the strength of the diaphragm. Coffee, soda, and chocolate contain xanthenes, which may explain why that morning cup of coffee helps you breathe a bit better. Examples of methylxanthines are:

- aminophylline (Truphylline)
- theophylline (Elixophyllin, Theo-24)

The side effects are similar to drinking too much coffee and include heartburn, stomach upset, headache, insomnia, irritability, tachycardia, and increased respiratory rate.

The use of methylxanthines requires titration to achieve the dose that delivers the desired effect while avoiding toxic levels. Blood should be drawn and levels monitored regularly to avoid serious side effects such as nausea and vomiting, low blood sugar levels, seizures, or heart irregularities. Methylxanthines should be used with caution because this type of bronchodilator can interact with a wide variety of medications and may increase your sense of nervousness or anxiety. Those who take methylxanthines should avoid drinking products that contain caffeine, such as coffee, soda, or tea.

Corticosteroids

Corticosteroids may be taken in an inhaled or oral form. The inhaled method is preferred because the medication targets the lungs and not the rest of the body, which reduces the occurrence of many side effects. Corticosteroids work to reduce the swelling and inflammation in your airways. They may also help decrease mucus production and decrease sensitivity to allergens and irritants. Sometimes they are combined with bronchodilators to provide better relief of symptoms. Corticosteroids take a while to begin working, so it is important to take them every day. Examples of corticosteroids are:

- beclomethasone (Beclovent, Vanceril, Qvar)
- triamcinolone (Azmacort)
- flunisolide (AeroBid)
- fluticasone (Flovent)
- budesonide (Pulmicort)

Corticosteroids should not be taken for fast relief. Do not stop taking them without consulting your health-care professional because serious side effects can occur. Always rinse your mouth thoroughly after taking your inhaled corticosteroid, preferably with an alcohol-based mouthwash. This helps prevent thrush, a yeast infection in the mouth. Thrush has been associated with inhaled corticosteroids.

Oral corticosteroids are often prescribed during an acute attack of COPD or for long-term maintenance. DO NOT STOP TAKING THESE WITHOUT CONSULTING YOUR HEALTH-CARE PROVIDER. The dose must be gradually tapered off to prevent serious side effects. Examples of oral corticosteroids are:

- prednisone (Orosone)
- prednisolone (Prelone)
- methylprednisolone (Medrol)

The side effects of taking oral corticosteroids are more severe than those of inhaled ones and include an increase in appetite, weight gain, stomach upset, headache, insomnia, and mood swings. The long-term effects of oral steroids include a weakened immune system, brittle bones, weight gain, fat deposits on the face and back, increased cholesterol levels, thinning skin, and cataracts.

Drug Combinations

There are many products that combine two medications into one easy-to-take treatment. Short-acting beta-agonists with anticholinergics include:

- albuterol sulfate + ipratroprium bromide = Duoneb or Combivent

Long-acting beta-agonists with corticosteroids include:

- salmeterol + fluticasone = Advair
- formoterol + budesonide = Symbicort

Expectorants

Expectorants are medications that help to break up thick mucus caused by infection or inflammation (*mucolytics*). They are administered orally or with a nebulizer. Examples of mucolytics are:

- acetylcysteine (Mucomyst): When nebulized, this medication has a familiar rotten egg odor. Sometimes Mucomyst can irritate your lungs. It should always be taken with a fast-acting bronchodilator. If your breathing becomes more difficult after a Mucomyst treatment, notify your health-care provider.

- guaifenesin: Taken orally, this medication is included in many over-the-counter cough and cold products such as Robitussin AC. It draws moisture into the lungs, thereby thinning mucus and making it easier to cough out. The side effects of guaifenesin include nausea, vomiting, and dry mouth.

Antibiotics

There are many types of antibiotics. Different antibiotics kill different bacteria. They are usually taken orally. If an infection is severe, they may be injected intravenously (thorough an IV catheter). Sometimes they may be combined with other medications. Your healthcare provider selects an antibiotic based on either a laboratory test or the type of bacteria he or she suspects is causing your infection.

It is important to take your antibiotics exactly as prescribed, even if you begin to feel better after a few days. Even though you feel better, there are still bacteria in your body. Completing the full course of antibiotics will prevent the infection from returning.

Leukotriene Modifiers

Taken orally, these medications help to decrease inflammation in a different way than steroids. Leukotrienes are chemicals released by the body that may trigger inflammation and bronchospasm. Leukotriene modifiers block the action of these chemicals to prevent attacks. They have not been properly tested for those with COPD but may be beneficial on a case-by-case basis.

Examples of leukotriene modifiers are:

- zafirlukast (Accolate)
- zileuton (Zyflo)
- montelukast (Singulair)

The side effects of leukotriene modifiers are dizziness, headache, fatigue, infection, and rash.

Benzodiazepines

Benzodiazepines may be prescribed to decrease feelings of panic or anxiety. These medications are prescribed with caution because their prolonged use may lead to physical dependence; however, if your life is crippled with anxiety and panic it is well worth the risk when used responsibly. Examples of benzodiazepines include:

- alprazolam (Xanax)
- diazepam (Valium)
- clonazepam (Klonopin)
- lorazepam (Ativan)

The side effects of benzodiazepines include dizziness, drowsiness, fatigue, or difficulty concentrating, although these side effects may disappear after your body becomes used to the medication. Use caution while operating hazardous equipment, motor vehicles, or any other activity that requires mental alertness until you know how the medication will affect you. Do not drink alcohol while taking benzodiazepines, because alcohol can enhance the medication's depressive effects on the nervous system, leading to a decreased respiratory drive.

Antidepressants

Feelings of depression are common when dealing with a chronic disease such as COPD. Depression can affect your body as well as your mind. If untreated, it can exacerbate your condition, leading to greater disability and more frequent hospitalizations. Unfortunately, few people with COPD seek treatment for depression and those who start treatment often do not follow through with treatment. This may be due to the feelings of hopelessness associated with chronic lung disease or to a negative social stigma about depression.

What you need to know is that depression is a treatable disorder no different from any other. A diabetic feels no shame when he takes his insulin and neither should you for seeking treatment for your feelings of depression. As a matter of fact, animal studies have shown that low oxygen levels may contribute to feelings of depression.

Symptoms of depression include the following:

- feelings of worthlessness, helplessness, or hopelessness
- sleeping more or less than usual
- eating more or less than usual

- difficulty concentrating or making decisions
- loss of interest in usual activities
- decrease or loss of sex drive
- avoiding others
- overwhelming feelings of sadness or grief
- loss of energy
- thoughts of death or suicide
- overwhelming feelings of guilt

If you have any of the above symptoms, tell your health-care provider and talk with him or her about your treatment options.

There are a wide variety of medications available to treat depression. They all work in different ways, and what helps one person may not help another. Sometimes two or three antidepressants must be tried before determining which one works best for you. If finances are tight, ask your doctor for samples until you are sure which medication he or she will ultimately prescribe. Don't give up. You deserve to feel better both physically and mentally. Examples of antidepressants are Paxil, Prozac, Cymbalta, and Effexor.

Side effects can vary. Ask your health-care provider or pharmacist about the side effects of your specific medication.

Medication Delivery

Inhaled medication can be administered in many forms, such as inhaled with a *metered-dose inhaler* (MDI), a *dry-powder inhaler* (DPI), or a small-volume nebulizer. Studies have shown that MDIs and nebulized medication can be equally effective in reducing or eliminating symptoms. However, some factors can diminish the effectiveness of MDIs, including the following:

Inability to coordinate puffs with breath: Those with arthritis, Parkinson's disease, or victims of stroke may have a difficult time depressing the dispenser. Nebulized medications may be more effective in these cases.

Inability to take a deep breath: If you are unable to take a deep breath, most of the medication delivered by the MDI will be deposited in the back of the throat and the upper airways, leaving the middle and lower airways unmedicated. Nebulized medications are delivered over a five- to ten-minute period of time, allowing the medication to gradually become deposited deep in the lower airways.

Inability to pay for MDIs: MDIs are expensive. Some insurance companies will not cover the cost of inhaled medication in MDI form but may cover these medications in the form used in a nebulizer.

Talk with your health-care provider if you are experiencing any of the issues listed above.

Metered-Dose Inhalers

Many medications come in metered-dose–inhaler form. The medication is in a canister that fits into an inhaler jacket. Often a tube called a spacer is attached to the inhaler. A spacer helps the medication move deeper into your lungs and prevents it from being deposited only in the mouth and throat. The use of a spacer also lessens certain side effects, such as hoarseness, sore throat, or unpleasant taste.

Steps for Using an Inhaler with a Spacer

In order to use an inhaler with a spacer, follow these steps:

1. Remove the caps from the inhaler and the spacer. Attach the spacer to the inhaler. Shake the inhaler well. Hold the inhaler with your index finger on the sprayer mechanism and your thumb around the spacer.

2. Breathe out normally through your nose. Place the opening of the spacer into your mouth, between your teeth. Close your lips around it. Press down once on the sprayer to spray one puff of medication into the spacer.

3. Slowly breathe in through your mouth as deeply as you can. This should take at least three to four seconds. If you

inhale too quickly, the spacer may whistle, reminding you to breathe in slower.

4. Hold your breath as you slowly count to ten. Then take the spacer out of your mouth. Pucker your lips like you are blowing out a candle. Breathe out slowly.

If you are prescribed more than one puff of medication at a time, wait at least one minute between puffs—unless told otherwise. Shake the inhaler and then repeat steps 2 through 4.

Using an Inhaler without a Spacer (Open-Mouth Method)

Although using a spacer is the preferred delivery method, some people choose not to use one. If you choose to proceed without using a spacer, the use of the open-mouth method is best. Apply the following steps for using an inhaler without a spacer:

1. Be sure to shake the inhaler well. Remove the cap and hold the inhaler upright.

2. Tilt your head backward and exhale all your air slowly.

3. Position the inhaler approximately 1 to 2 inches in front of your open mouth.

4. Firmly press down on the canister as you begin to inhale.

5. Breathe in for a count of five.

6. Hold your breath as you slowly count to ten.

7. Slowly exhale.

Wait at least one minute and repeat all of the above steps if more than one puff is prescribed.

When to Replace Your Inhaler

Each inhaler contains only a certain number of puffs. Some inhalers have counters, while others do not. To be sure you get enough medication when you need it, keep track of how many puffs you use. Here is a tip to help you calculate when you should replace your inhaler:

- Find the number on the canister that tells you how many puffs it contains.

- Divide this number by how many puffs you are told to use in one day. This gives you the number of days your medication should last.

- Use your calendar to determine the date your medication will run out. Mark the date on your canister and on your calendar.

Be sure to replace your inhaler before you run out of medication. Also note that your medication will run out sooner if you use your inhaler more often than planned.

Cleaning Your Inhaler

Always keep the cap on your inhaler when not in use. Without the cap, dust, debris, and even objects such as coins can get inside and be inhaled into your lungs. Clean your inhaler at least once a week to prevent the medication from building up inside the canister or causing blockage. Here are some tips for cleaning your inhaler:

- Remove the canister and mouthpiece from the dispenser and set them aside. Do not wash or immerse the canister.

- Wash the dispenser by holding it under warm running water for thirty seconds. Shake out the excess water, place it on a paper towel, and let the dispenser dry overnight.

- Replace the canister and mouthpiece when the dispenser is dry.

The "New" Inhalers

Due to environmental and public health concerns, the FDA now requires the replacement of CFC (chlorofluorocarbon) propellants, which have been proven to cause damage to the ozone, with HFA (*hydrofluoroalkane*) propellants in inhalers as well as other aerosolized products.

Many people using the "new" inhalers have expressed concern about their effectiveness. Although HFA inhalers have a finer mist and may taste or feel differently, they work just as effectively as the "old" inhalers. The spray is less forceful, but use of a spacer with an HFA inhaler, as with any propellant inhaler, will help capture the medication and deposit it more effectively in your lungs. If you still have concerns, consult your health-care provider.

Dry-Powder Inhalers

Dry-powder inhalers (DPIs) deliver a measured dose of medication in a dry powder form. Some DPIs deliver only one medication and others deliver a combination of medications.

The technique for use of a DPI is different from that of a metered-dose inhaler. Because there is no propellant, it is important to inhale the medication quickly and deeply. Be sure to hold your breath for a count of five before exhaling. There are several styles of dry-powder inhalers. Be sure to carefully read the directions for use. If you have any questions, ask your pharmacist or health-care provider for more information about proper usage.

Primatene Mist Inhalers

Primatene Mist is an over-the-counter product that should be *avoided* by those with COPD. Its primary ingredient is epinephrine (adrenaline), and while it does act as a bronchodilator, it is also a strong stimulant of the heart and can cause a dangerous increase in blood pressure and heart rate that can lead to heart attack or stroke. It may also cause seizures, tremors, or extreme irritability. Albuterol sulfate is always the better choice because it has a lower risk of serious side effects. If you are currently using a Primatene Mist inhaler, consult your health-care provider about better options.

Nebulizers

A nebulizer is a device used to change liquid medication into an aerosolized form. The nebulizer consists of a medication cup, a "tee" piece, a mouthpiece, and tubing. The tubing is attached to a small air compressor. When the air travels through the tube and reaches the cup, it breaks the liquid down into an aerosol that you inhale. It is important to complete the entire treatment for maximum effectiveness.

After each treatment, the nebulizer should be taken apart and rinsed in running water. Every day, the nebulizer should be disassembled, washed in warm soapy water, rinsed, and allowed to air dry. Once a week, the disassembled parts should be soaked in a warm water/white vinegar solution for decontamination. Use one part vinegar to four parts of water. Soak for thirty minutes, rinse, and allow to air dry.

Oxygen

Oxygen is considered a drug when prescribed by your health-care provider to treat low blood oxygen levels (hypoxia). It is critical that your oxygen levels be tested at rest, with exercise, and at night. If low blood oxygen levels are caught early, continuous home oxygen therapy may be prevented or delayed.

Normal blood oxygen levels are usually 90 to 100 percent. Health-care providers typically prescribe supplemental home oxygen when your blood oxygen level is less than 88 percent. It is important to use your oxygen exactly as prescribed. If left untreated, low oxygen levels can cause the following problems:

- decreased mental function
- decreased exercise tolerance
- fatigue
- headaches
- decreased life expectancy
- decreased quality of life
- quicker progression of the disease
- development of heart disease
- increased risk for stroke

Supplemental home oxygen is not a death warrant. It is simply another medication used to treat the symptoms of COPD. Everyone needs oxygen. People with low oxygen levels just need a little bit extra than those with healthy lungs. At 2 lpm (liters per minute) you are receiving approximately 27 percent oxygen. That is just 6 percent more than those with healthy lungs. But that 6 percent can make all the difference in how you feel and how your body functions. Use the chart in Table 4.1 to determine the percentage of extra oxygen your body needs:

TABLE 4.1: Concentration of Oxygen as Determined by Liter Flow

Liter Flow per Minute (lpm)	Fraction of Inspired Oxygen (FIO_2)
1	24 percent
2	27 percent
3	30 percent
4	33 percent
5	36 percent

Supplemental Oxygen Myths

Myth: I just need a "whiff" now and then and I am fine.
Truth: The body cannot "store up" oxygen like you would store gasoline in your car's fuel tank. The "whiff" will briefly increase your oxygen levels, but they will quickly return to a lower level once you remove the oxygen.

Myth: I don't want to become addicted to oxygen so I don't use it very often.
Truth: We are all "addicted" to oxygen. No one can live without it.

Myth: Once I am on oxygen, I can never leave home.
Truth: There are many lightweight, portable oxygen systems that allow for a full and active lifestyle.

Myth: I feel fine without my oxygen, so I don't need to use it.
Truth: The human body is an amazing thing. It can adapt to diverse conditions, such as low oxygen levels, but not for long. Although you may feel fine, serious and long-term damage may be occurring to your brain, heart, and other vital organs when your oxygen levels are low.

Home Oxygen Equipment

There are three common ways of providing home oxygen therapy: oxygen concentrators, compressed gas, and liquid oxygen.

■ Oxygen Concentrators

An oxygen concentrator is an electrically powered machine that separates room air into nitrogen and oxygen. The nitrogen is discarded, while the pure oxygen is stored, concentrated, and delivered at 90 to 95 percent purity. If using an oxygen concentrator, you should advise your electric power company in order to get priority service if there is a power failure. Concentrators are a good choice if you need oxygen all the time or while sleeping.

ALARMS

The oxygen concentrator has alarms to alert you to a power failure or an equipment malfunction. If the alarm sounds, follow these steps:

1. If you are on continuous oxygen, be sure to have your backup tank ready and use it if it becomes necessary.

2. Check to see if the machine is plugged into the wall outlet.

3. If plugged into a wall outlet that is controlled by a wall switch, make sure the switch is in the on position.

4. Check to see if you have power to your house. There may be a power failure. If there is a power failure, turn the machine off to stop the alarm.

5. Check your fuses or circuit breakers to determine if one has blown.

6. Make sure your oxygen tubing is not kinked. Kinked tubing creates back pressure that may cause the alarm to sound.

7. If you have a humidifier, take it off and connect your oxygen tubing directly to the machine. Humidifiers can become clogged, causing the machine to alarm. If this works, replace the clogged humidifier with a new one.

If none of these steps work, turn the machine off and contact your oxygen supplier to send someone to fix or replace your machine.

■ Compressed Gas

Oxygen is stored under pressure in a cylinder equipped with a regulator that controls the flow of the gas. An oxygen-conserving device may be attached to the system to avoid waste and increase the lifetime of your cylinder. This is a good choice if you don't use oxygen all the time.

■ Liquid Oxygen

Oxygen is stored as a very cold liquid in a vessel similar to a thermos. When released, the liquid converts to a gas and you breathe it just like you would with compressed gas. This is a good choice if you are very active but need to wear oxygen all the time.

Oxygen Safety

Although not flammable, oxygen does support combustion. This means that oxygen can make a fire burn hotter and faster. Stay at least ten feet away from gas stoves, lighted fireplaces, candles, and other sources of heat or open flame.

Serious burns have occurred to those who smoke cigarettes while wearing their oxygen. Do not smoke or allow others to smoke near you when using oxygen.

Use water-based lubricants to moisten your lips and nostrils. Never use an oil-based product like Vaseline. A chemical reaction between oil-based products and oxygen can cause serious burning of the skin.

Oxygen Delivery Devices

If you are prescribed oxygen to treat COPD, there are three main delivery systems. The device you use will often depend on the level of oxygen being administered. Some commonly used devices are nasal cannulas, face masks, and oxygen reservoir devices.

Nasal cannula: This is a plastic tube that is inserted into the nose. Sometimes new cannulas have an odor that is offensive. Many people describe this odor as a "plastic" or "chemical" smell. If you find this to be the case, open the package and let the cannula "air out" before use.

Oxygen mask: If you use oxygen at 6 lpm or greater, the flow of oxygen though the cannula may cause drying of the nose. A mask that fits over the nose and mouth may be more comfortable; however, it can be used only at greater than 6 lpm or you will be unable to clear exhaled carbon dioxide from the mask, potentially causing respiratory failure.

Oxygen reservoir device: These devices are often called "oxymizers." They typically employ a pendant or nosepiece that "collects" oxygen and can provide much higher amounts of oxygen at lower liter flows than a nasal cannula can.

CHAPTER 5

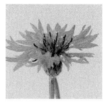

Alternative Therapies

As you have learned, there is no cure for COPD. However, there are treatments and surgical procedures that you may want to consider. All have strict criteria and come with varying degrees of risk, but they may help those who desire to enjoy a better quality of life.

Noninvasive Positive Pressure Respiratory Assist Devices

The use of a noninvasive positive pressure device is controversial but may help those with severe end-stage COPD or those with chronic carbon dioxide retention. It is typically used while sleeping. When using a noninvasive positive pressure device, your breathing is supported by a machine that pushes air into your lungs when you inhale through a snug mask that fits either over your nose or over your nose and mouth. This *inspiratory positive airway pressure* (IPAP) helps fill your lungs, thereby allowing you to breath deeper with less work. When you exhale, an *expiratory positive airway pressure* (EPAP) remains that helps to splint your smaller airways open and relieve the air trapping that causes carbon dioxide levels to build. Some machines have a backup rate that will deliver breaths if you experience apnea (cessation of breathing for short periods of time) or hypoventilation (small, shallow breathing that does not allow for gas exchange).

Apnea or hypoventilation with oxygen desaturation is common for those with COPD. Not only does this abnormal breathing pattern disrupt sleep, but it can also worsen respiratory muscle function. Noninvasive positive pressure devices help to support your breathing while resting the breathing muscles to allow for better sleep and more energy.

Insurance coverage varies; however, most companies follow the Medicare guidelines. To qualify for coverage with Medicare you must:

- Have a prescription from your doctor.

- Get an ABG. Your PCO_2 must be greater than or equal to 52 mmHg while awake and breathing normally. An ABG drawn during a flare-up would not be acceptable.

- Have an overnight oximetry test either in the hospital or in your home. Your oxygen saturation level must go below 88 percent for at least five minutes while using at least 2 lpm of supplemental oxygen. If you use a higher liter flow, the test must be done while using your usual amount of oxygen.

If you meet the above criteria, a noninvasive positive pressure device should be covered by your insurance. The machine is supplied by most home oxygen providers and will require a respiratory therapist to help you become comfortable with the machine and its use.

After sixty-one days of use, Medicare requires a signed document from you, as well as your doctor, stating that you are using the machine for at least four hours in a twenty-four–hour period and that you are benefitting from its use. Medicare will then continue coverage at its usual rate of 80 percent. Secondary insurance, if available, should cover the remainder.

Those who have had success in using noninvasive positive pressure devices report having more energy, less shortness of breath, and improved lung function.

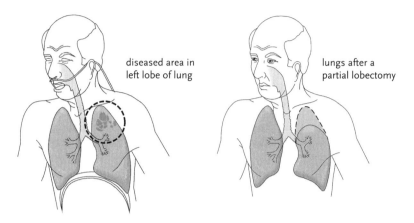

diseased area in
left lobe of lung

lungs after a
partial lobectomy

FIGURE 5.1: Lung volume reduction surgery

Lung Volume Reduction Surgery

Lung volume reduction surgery (LVRS) is a procedure that removes diseased lung tissue so that the healthy tissue that remains can work more efficiently. Up to 30 percent of the lungs may be removed (see Figure 5.1).

LVRS does not cure COPD, but it can improve quality of life by decreasing shortness of breath, increasing lung function, and improving energy and mobility. The best candidates for this surgery are those with severe emphysema in the upper lung lobes who are otherwise healthy and have made little or no progress in a formal pulmonary rehabilitation program.

As with all surgical procedures, there are risks involved, including scarring, serious infection, and death. Medicare will typically cover this procedure if you have:

- emphysema
- quit smoking at least four months prior to the procedure
- no history of coronary artery bypass graft surgery or some other heart complications

Talk with your health-care provider if you are interested in more information about lung volume reduction surgery.

Lung Transplantation

The transplant of one or both lungs is typically a treatment of last resort reserved for those with severe end-stage lung disease. Although the procedure might not lengthen your life, it can make your remaining years more enjoyable by improving lung function and your ability to exercise, and decreasing your shortness of breath.

Waiting for a donor can be a lengthy process but living donors have been used. This procedure should not be considered lightly, because it has serious risks, such as rejection, death, and infection. Those who receive a lung transplant must take immunosuppressant drugs for the rest of their lives, thereby increasing their risk of infection.

To be considered for lung transplantation, you must:

- be less than sixty-five years of age and have end-stage lung disease
- be ambulatory
- be at an ideal body weight
- have hypercapnia with associated pulmonary hypertension
- have an $FEV_1 < 20$ percent of normally predicted

Many insurance companies will cover lung transplantation on a case-by-case basis. Talk with your health-care provider if you meet the above criteria and would like more information.

Nebulized Morphine

Morphine is an opioid-based narcotic used frequently to reduce the symptoms of shortness of breath and pain. It is typically given through your IV while in the hospital, or it may be prescribed and taken orally for chronic pain.

Nebulized morphine is inhaled through a small-volume nebulizer, just like albuterol. While there is much controversy surrounding this practice, it does seem to alleviate shortness of breath for those with end-stage lung disease. When inhaled, it targets opioid receptors in the lungs, acting quickly to reduce *dyspnea* and pain with less of a sedative effect on the rest of the body. This may be a viable option for those in hospice or as a palliative (comfort) care measure while in the hospital.

Naturopathic Remedies

There are many products advertised in magazines, on television, and on the Internet that claim to add "extra" oxygen to the body, reduce or eliminate your symptoms, and even cure COPD. As you now know, there, unfortunately, is no cure for COPD, nor can you "top off" your oxygen levels as if your lungs were a tank of gasoline. However, there have been limited studies conducted with some nutritional supplements that seem to help certain symptoms associated with COPD.

Omega-3 Fatty Acids

Omega-3 fatty acids are unsaturated fatty acids that seem to decrease shortness of breath and the rate of lung function decline, as well as to increase the exercise capacity for those with COPD. However, the benefits don't end there. There is strong evidence to suggest that an adequate intake of omega-3 fatty acids may lower triglycerides, slow the buildup of plaque in the veins and arteries, and help to lower blood pressure. Studies also show a reduction in the risk of death from a heart attack, dangerous heart arrhythmias, and stroke for those with known heart disease.

Omega-3 fatty acids are important to the human body. They can be found in varying degrees in many species of cold-water, oily fish; English walnuts; and a variety of vegetable oils, such as canola, flax, linseed, soybean, and olive. However, omega-3 fatty acids can react with certain prescription medications, especially those affecting the heart, blood pressure, and blood sugar, and/or blood thinners such as Coumadin. Talk to your health-care provider before taking omega-3 supplements.

Beta-Carotene

Beta-carotene is a strong antioxidant found in colorful fruits and vegetables, such as green plants, carrots, sweet potatoes, squash, spinach, apricots, and green peppers. Think dark green, yellow, red, or orange when in the produce section of your grocery store.

Experts recommend five servings of foods rich in beta-carotene per day. The body only needs approximately 2 mg of beta-carotene per day, so healthy eating may be all you need to reap the benefits of this antioxidant.

Limited studies have suggested that beta-carotene can reduce shortness of breath and episodes of acute bronchitis. However, supplements may actually increase the risk of cancer in smokers, so if you are still smoking, this may be something you stay away from in large doses.

Ginseng

Ginseng is a root that is widely used in Chinese medicine. It is thought to improve lung function and exercise tolerance for those with COPD.

Chinese practitioners recommend taking 100 to 200 mg/day of American or Asian ginseng for two to three weeks, and then taking a one- to two-week break. Do not take more than 1 g of dry root daily because it can cause seizures, confusion, or problems with bleeding when taken in very high doses. Although ginseng is generally well tolerated, it can interact with many medications such as insulin, antihypertensives, painkillers, or certain antidepressants.

Always talk with your health-care provider before taking any herbs or supplements. Also, add any herbs or supplements you use to your medication list, so if you are hospitalized, the interactions can be considered before starting treatment.

CHAPTER 6

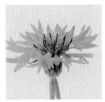

Dealing with Your Emotions

How many of these statements describe how you feel right now?

- COPD is the worst possible thing that could ever happen to me.
- I'll never be able to do what I want to do again.
- No one understands what I am going through.
- Why bother trying? I am going to die soon anyway.
- It's my fault this happened. I deserve to suffer.

All of the above feelings are normal. Being diagnosed with a chronic illness can be devastating. Even if you have been experiencing symptoms for a long period of time, learning that you have COPD may trigger thoughts of anger, fear, and denial. Suddenly you are faced with the potential loss of health, mobility, and independence. These losses are no different from the loss of anything else of great importance in your life. It is normal to move through a wide range of emotions when experiencing grief due to loss. This emotional journey is called the process of grieving.

The Grieving Process

Major losses in life can make us feel alone, depressed, and withdrawn. These feelings are normal and an important part of what professionals call the grieving process. Everyone needs a period of reflection before he or she can move forward.

Grief is a natural response to the loss of something important to you. The loss may be your spouse, your job, your financial stability, or your health. The grieving process helps you to move through the painful emotional stages that come with grief and eventually come to terms with your loss.

The grieving process was first described in 1969 by Elisabeth Kübler-Ross, a psychiatrist who worked closely with the terminally ill. She identified what has come to be known as the "five stages of grief." While originally used to describe the feelings of those facing a terminal illness, it is now understood that any important loss in life can cause a person to grieve. These stages are not a rigid timetable but rather a guide to help people understand that these emotions are normal and healthy. You may not experience all of the stages, or you may move back and forth between two or three. Just know that your goal is to work through these stages by feeling your emotions, by asking for help, and ultimately by learning to accept your condition. Only then will you be ready to work with your limitations, take control of your symptoms, and improve your quality of life.

Keep in mind that there is no timetable for grief. Everyone grieves differently. It doesn't matter if your neighbor was over the loss of her husband in three months or your family believes that you should be moving on. Grieving is a very individual process and depends on many factors, such as your personality, your coping skills, your life experiences, and the nature of the loss. Just know that getting stuck in one of these emotional stages can be detrimental to your mental and physical health. There are some things you can do to help you work through your feelings.

The Five Stages of Grief

1. Denial: "There is nothing wrong with me. I am fine."
Shock and denial are common when one is first diagnosed with a chronic disease. Many people describe feeling disconnected from their body or just, plain numb. You may have trouble sleeping or

feel restless or alone. Keeping connected with supportive friends or family is important in this stage.

2. Anger: "Why is this happening to me?"

Anger is the number-one feeling for many suffering a chronic disease. You may feel angry at yourself, your doctor, your spouse, or even at God. It may seem unfair that you have been diagnosed with a disease that will rob you of a future you have envisioned. Sometimes anger spills over and becomes blame. This is an easy emotion to become stuck in and may require the most work to get through. Setting positive goals seems to be the best antidote for anger.

3. Bargaining: "Make this go away and I'll go to church every Sunday."

Most people would promise almost anything to make their COPD go away. When you are in this emotional stage, you may feel as if you can "make a deal" with God, promising something in return for a cure. When a cure does not happen, you may feel angry or depressed, thereby triggering a different emotional stage. This is okay and it is part of the grieving process.

4. Depression: "Why do anything at all? I am just going to die anyway."

Depression associated with grief may come and go. It may be triggered by certain events, such as going to the doctor or on the anniversary of your diagnosis. If depression becomes severe or prolonged, it may be necessary to seek counseling to help you through these difficult times.

5. Acceptance: "I've come to terms with my illness and am ready to move forward."

This is the point where you have come to accept that your disease is a part of who you are and you become ready to deal with it constructively. You have learned new skills and are willing to make changes in your lifestyle to cope with the limitations of your disease. You know that you don't have to give up anything to do what you enjoy. You just need to learn new ways of doing the things you have always done and can continue to do.

Coping with Grief and Loss

After receiving your diagnosis, you will need to find ways to cope with your sense of loss and the grief you feel. Don't be afraid to ask friends and family for their help and support during this time.

Get Support

Even if you don't have anyone in your immediate family to help you through this stage, there are many other places where you can obtain support. Friends, churches, and support groups can provide you with the help you need by connecting you with resources and by offering emotional support through the difficult times by reminding you that you are not a disease—but a person.

Take Care of Yourself

When wrapped up in the grieving process, it is easy to forget to take care of yourself. You may not feel like taking a shower in the morning or even getting out of bed. However, the simple process of getting up and getting ready for the day can help to remind you that every day is a new opportunity for growth, for change, and for joy. Know that the mind and body are connected. When you feel better physically, you will feel better emotionally as well. Eat well, exercise, get good sleep, and do not use drugs or alcohol to numb your pain. The only way to move through it is to feel it.

Face, Feel, and Express Your Emotions

To make progress toward accepting your disease and learning to adapt, you must face your feelings. Facing these feelings can be a very painful process, but ignoring or avoiding your feelings will only make things worse in the long term. Not only does avoidance make it harder and take longer to move through the grieving process, but it can also lead to health problems, self-medication with drugs or alcohol, and/or anxiety and severe depression.

Ask for Help

Asking for help is not a sign of weakness. There is nothing noble about unnecessary isolation or suffering. There are always people willing to help, not because they pity you but because they care for you. Don't ever be afraid to ask for help. Everyone needs help from time to time in their life. Ask yourself: Wouldn't you be willing to help a friend? Why wouldn't your friends or family be willing to help you?

Getting Stuck

You know you are stuck in an emotional stage when it begins to negatively affect how you manage your disease. If you find it difficult to move out of an emotional stage, seek outside help from a counselor or therapist. Ask your doctor or other health-care provider for a referral if you are unsure as to where to go, especially if you find yourself stuck in one of the emotional stages listed below. Your health-care provider will be happy to steer you in the right direction.

Denial

As you have learned, shock and denial are common reactions when one is diagnosed with a chronic illness. However, when denial is extended over a long period of time, it will lead to poor disease management. Harmful denial includes not taking your medication as prescribed, denying the need for help from outside support systems, and/or overdoing by ignoring your feelings of shortness of breath and pushing your body beyond its limits. Unresolved or prolonged denial may not only increase the severity of your symptoms, but it may also speed up the progression of your disease.

Anger

It is common to be angry when you are diagnosed with COPD. You may not be able to be as active as you once were. You may feel that you have lost your independence. Sometimes you may feel angry at yourself. At other times you may feel angry at those around you. It is okay to be angry. Anger is part of the grieving process. Prolonged anger, however, can be detrimental to your physical as well as mental health. One of the best things you can to do to move away from anger is to set some realistic goals and begin working toward them. Not only will these goals help you to gain a greater sense of control over your life, they will allow you to focus on the progress that you are making rather than what you have lost.

Blame

Blame and anger are intimately related. You may blame yourself for COPD. You may blame others. Blame is another unhealthy reaction to adversity. When blaming yourself or others, you may never get around to the work of correcting your behavior because you are busy punishing those whom you perceive to be at fault.

Unhealthy: "I smoked and caused my COPD; therefore, I am a terrible person."

Better: "Perhaps I really did cause my COPD by smoking. That was a mistake. Humans frequently make mistakes; I am definitely human. The past is the past. Now I need to move forward and discover what I can do now to feel better and deal better."

Depression

Feelings of depression are basically feelings of sadness that go along with a loss. It is okay to grieve for your losses. They are significant to you. However, as with prolonged anger, prolonged depression is unhealthy. If depression is affecting your ability to manage your disease, get help! Talk to your health-care professional. There are more options than ever for treating depression.

Signs of Depression

- feeling worthless, helpless, or hopeless
- sleeping more or less than usual
- eating more or less than usual
- difficulty concentration or making decisions
- loss of interest in activities
- decreased sex drive
- avoiding others
- overwhelming feelings of sadness or grief
- loss of energy

- thoughts of death or suicide
- feelings of guilt

Fear

Fear is a normal reaction to change. You may fear losing control of your life. You may fear death or the thought of life with a chronic disease. These are rational fears that can be reduced or eliminated in many ways. Joining a support group, working through this book, gathering information—these are all ways to eliminate fear. However, not all fears are rational. Irrational fears and thoughts can cloud your mind and interfere with your ability to manage your disease. Consider the statements below. Face your irrational fears and replace them with facts.

Irrational fear: "If I get short of breath in public, it will be a disaster. I will never be able to show my face in public again."

Better: "So what if I get short of breath? Like I care what strangers think. I may get short of breath, but I'm not going to let it stop me from enjoying the things I like to do."

Anxiety

Anxiety and panic are commonly felt by those with COPD—and with good reason. When the body senses a low oxygen level, it releases chemicals that increase the heart and respiratory rate. This reaction is sometimes described as the fight-or-flight response. Unfortunately, this response can lead to panic and a vicious cycle begins, as you can see in Figure 6.1 on the next page.

Jeannie talks about her anxiety:

"Every time my daughter-in-law comes to visit, I become very anxious. The last visit was particularly bad. She was trying to convince me to move in with her and my son and I was having none of that. The more she talked the harder it became to breathe. By the time she left, I couldn't catch my breath. I sat there on the couch, huffing and puffing, sure I was going to die. The worst part was feeling so helpless."

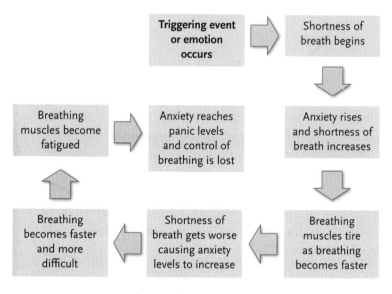

FIGURE 6.1: *The cycle of anxiety*

There are several ways to break this cycle before you reach the panic level. Two methods that work particularly well when you are short of breath are focused relaxation and controlled, pursed-lip breathing. Both methods are covered in Chapter 8.

CHAPTER 7

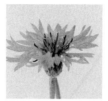

Your Flare-up
Action Plan

Flare-ups (exacerbations) of your COPD can be frightening as well as life threatening if not caught early. Flare-ups seem to happen to some people more often than to others. Frequent flare-ups can severely affect your quality of life. It can take a long time to recover from a flare-up, and one may cause further lung damage.

What Is a Flare-up?

A flare-up, or exacerbation, can best be described as the point when your COPD symptoms become so bad that you require emergent care and possibly hospitalization. It can be brought on by allergies, by infections such as a cold or the flu, or by simply being worn down by excess stress or activity.

The process usually begins with coldlike symptoms as inflammation in the airways increases, making them more sensitive to irritants. This leads to airway constriction and increased mucus production, causing a cough and an increase in shortness of breath. Oxygen levels drop and carbon dioxide levels increase due to trapped air in the lungs. This condition can lead to *acute respiratory failure* and the need for emergency care.

Signs and Symptoms of an Exacerbation

Ignoring or disregarding the following signs and symptoms of exacerbation can lead to acute respiratory failure:

- new or worsening shortness of breath
- increased mucus
- blood, unusual or foul odor, or yellow or green mucus production
- new or increased wheezing
- tiredness
- sore throat
- fever
- poor response to bronchodilators

Acute respiratory failure means that your lungs can no longer provide enough oxygen to your body nor can the lungs remove carbon dioxide effectively. Without emergency treatment, this condition will lead to death. Luckily, there are many things you can do to decrease your risk for an exacerbation of your COPD.

Identify Your Triggers

You have already learned how your lungs work and how important it is to take your medication as prescribed. Learning to identify triggers to flare-ups will allow you to better manage your COPD.

Triggers are those things that make it more difficult to breathe. The obvious triggers are often the ones that are physical, such as allergens, irritants, or infection. Less obvious triggers are emotional ones, such as stress or anxiety.

Take a moment to think about the physical things in your environment that cause you to become short of breath. Some common allergens and irritants are listed in Figure 7.1. Do any of these irritants seem to make your breathing worse?

Do you find yourself avoiding the physical things that make your breathing worse? If you are avoiding them, then congratulations. This is the first step toward feeling better. If you are unsure of what

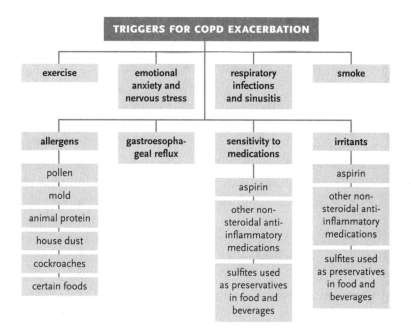

FIGURE 7.1: *Common triggers for COPD exacerbation*

triggers your shortness of breath, try keeping a daily log to keep track of what seems to make your symptoms worse. Keeping an accurate record makes it easier to pinpoint what triggers your shortness of breath. Taking care to avoid these things will have you breathing easier in no time.

Hand Washing

Hand washing is your first and most important line of defense against infection. Many viruses can survive as long as forty-eight hours outside the human body, lurking on surfaces like doorknobs, kitchen counters, and bathroom sinks. Using the technique below will ensure you wash your hands effectively:

- Wet your hands in warm, running water.
- Add soap. Rub your hands vigorously and thoroughly. Make sure you don't forget the back of your hands and around your nails.

- Wash for at least twenty seconds. Count slowly to twenty to be sure you wash long enough.
- Rinse your hands well and leave the water running.
- Dry your hands with a paper towel, and then use the paper towel to turn off the faucet. If you are in a public bathroom, use the same towel to open the door handle when you exit.

Alcohol-Based Sanitizers

Alcohol-based sanitizers work just as well as soap and water as long as your hands are not visibly soiled. Squirt about half a teaspoon into the palm of your hand and rub your hands together vigorously until they are dry. Make sure your hand sanitizer is at least 60 percent alcohol, because water-based sanitizers are not as effective. Today, you can purchase little bottles that fit conveniently in your purse or pocket at many types of stores.

Get Your Flu Shot

The Centers for Disease Control (CDC) recommends an annual flu shot if you:

- are over age fifty
- have a chronic illness like COPD
- live in an environment in which you are in close contact with others at risk, such as a nursing home or assisted-living facility

The flu shot is a vaccine that contains an inactive, or "dead," form of the flu virus. Because it is inactive, you cannot get the flu from the vaccine. When the vaccine is injected, your immune system creates antibodies that will attack and defend against the "live" virus should you be exposed later. It takes about two weeks to be fully protected, so avoid people with the flu during that time period.

Generally, you should get a flu shot as soon as the vaccine becomes available, usually in September or October. Keep in mind that flu season runs from October to May. Side effects resulting from a flu shot include pain, redness, or swelling at the injection site; low-grade fever; or muscle aches. These effects should pass in two to three days. Getting a flu shot may decrease your risk of serious illness or death by up to 50 percent. The shots are widely available and can be obtained at your doctor's office, pharmacies, local senior centers, and most hospitals. Talk with your doctor or check your local newspaper to see where flu shots are available.

Get a Pneumonia Shot

Pneumonia is the leading vaccine-preventable death in the United States. Because pneumonia has become resistant to many common antibiotics, it is more important than ever to be vaccinated. The pneumonia shot protects against twenty-three types of the disease. The CDC recommends pneumonia shots to those:

- over age sixty-five
- with a chronic disease like COPD
- living in a high-risk environment, such as a nursing home or assisted-living facility

The side effects resulting from a pneumonia shot are similar to those of the flu shot and should disappear within a couple of days. Talk to your doctor to see if and when a pneumonia shot is right for you.

More Tips to Avoid Exacerbation

In addition to identifying your triggers, practicing good hygiene, and getting a flu and pneumonia shot, the following tips will also help you avoid exacerbation:

Avoid crowds: Especially during cold and flu season. Shop earlier or later than peak hours and stay out of packed theaters.

Exercise, eat a balanced diet, and sleep: Maintaining a healthy immune system requires care. Don't let yourself become run down, worn out, or too tired.

Keep lungs clear of mucus: Excess mucus in your lungs makes breathing more difficult and provides bacteria with an ideal breeding ground. Use the techniques described in Chapter 8 to help clear the mucus from your lungs.

Avoid allergens: Minimize or eliminate your exposure to allergens. Take your allergy medications as prescribed.

Learn to listen to your body: If you have new or worsening symptoms, your body is trying to tell you that something is wrong. Just as chest pain alerts you of a heart attack, an increase in symptoms may be warning you of impending respiratory failure. Taking care of yourself promptly will decrease the risk of a situation turning into a major medical event, costing you money, health, and perhaps your life.

Prepare

Despite your best efforts, you may still have flare-ups. Why is that? Due to COPD, your lungs have lost some of their ability to fight infection. They may be more sensitive to changes in the environment. You must be alert to certain changes in your lungs so that you can catch the irritation, inflammation, or infection early and avoid the need for hospitalization. You must also develop an action plan based on your particular symptoms. Many times doctors will prescribe prednisone or antibiotics for you to have ready to use if you think a flare-up is happening. Call your doctor if you experience any of the following warning signs so that you can start treatment as soon as possible:

- increasing shortness of breath
- increased coughing that produces mucus
- change in mucus color, thickness, or odor, or mucus that is blood-streaked
- swelling in ankles, feet, or legs
- new or worsening wheezing
- loss of energy or progressive weakness

- working harder to breathe
- feelings of depression or hopelessness
- fever
- faster breathing or pulse rate
- inability to cough out mucus

Emergency Treatment

Flare-ups happen. Perhaps yours progressed rapidly or was unresponsive to treatment at home. Whatever the reason, it is critical to seek emergency treatment if you experience any of the following symptoms:

- rapid increase in shortness of breath
- feeling drowsy or less alert
- shortness of breath at rest with no relief
- breathing faster than 25 breaths per minute
- pulse greater than 110 beats per minute
- nail bed and lips are blue (if not normally blue)
- using shoulder or neck muscles to breath

What to Expect

It is normal to be frightened when you feel as if you cannot breathe. Knowing what to expect can help relieve the stress and anxiety of a hospital visit.

■ In the Emergency Room

Once you are in the emergency room, the health-care provider will order a variety of tests. An ABG may be drawn to determine if you have enough oxygen in your blood and are eliminating carbon dioxide effectively. A chest X ray (CXR) may be taken to see if you have pneumonia. An electrocardiogram (EKG) may be performed to make sure your heart is beating correctly and to rule out a cardiac reason (such as a heart attack) for your shortness of breath. Blood will be drawn to check for infection, dehydration, and other problems.

One or more IVs may be started and the doctor may order fluids to keep you hydrated, steroids such as Solu-Medrol to decrease the inflammation in your lungs, and antibiotics if infection is suspected. Medication delivered directly into your veins through an IV will work much more quickly and efficiently than if taken orally. You may receive medication to help decrease your anxiety and/or panic and breathing treatments may be given frequently or continuously to help relax your lungs.

If these therapies fail to increase your lung function and decrease your shortness of breath, advanced treatment may be considered. One method of treatment that works 70 percent of the time is called noninvasive positive pressure ventilation (NIPPV). This form of ventilation is designed to help you breathe easier, increase your oxygen levels, and decrease your carbon dioxide levels until your body has responded to the medications your doctor has ordered.

NIPPV supports your breathing by delivering air and oxygen under pressure to your lungs through a mask that fits over your mouth and nose. The snug seal required for it to work effectively can be difficult to tolerate at first, but it is definitely worth any initial discomfort, because the next step is *intubation*. The doctor may order antianxiety medication or sedation to make NIPPV easier to tolerate.

Intubation is a procedure in which a tube is place down in the throat to deliver air and oxygen to the lungs. The tube is attached to a mechanical ventilator (respirator). This machine delivers breaths to your lungs until you are able to breathe effectively on your own. Intubation requires specialized care in the intensive care unit. It is difficult for many people with COPD to withdraw from mechanical ventilation because it can increase the risk for secondary infections and can cause weakness of the breathing muscles.

After a prolonged hospital stay for an exacerbation of COPD, you may require the services of physical, occupational, or speech therapists. You may need to rebuild your strength and relearn the activities of daily living. Having a tube in your throat for an extended period of time may cause damage resulting in swallowing difficulties. A speech therapist can ensure that you are able to swallow without inhaling food or water into your lungs.

End-of-Life Choices

No one likes to think about dying, but the reality is we are all going to do it whether we are ready or not. By preparing beforehand, you can make choices about your medical care before an emergency occurs that will affect your quality of life as well as the dying process itself.

Talk with Your Family

Make sure your family knows your wishes in the event of an emergency. Discuss which medical treatment you do or do not want. Remember that your family will be speaking for you when you cannot. Let them know your wishes regarding:

Intubation and mechanical ventilation: Do you want it? For how long?

Resuscitation: If your heart stops, do you want chest compressions and medications delivered in an attempt to restart your heart? Chest compressions can be brutal for the elderly and those with COPD because the bones of your ribs and chest may be broken in the process.

Tube feeding: Do you want a tube placed in your stomach to feed your body in the event that you cannot eat? Do you want one temporarily or permanently?

Comfort care: Would you rather not be aggressively resuscitated but be made comfortable in your final days or hours?

Advance Directives

An advance directive is a written record outlining your desires in the event of a life-threatening emergency. It should be completed and kept on file with your doctor and the hospital you use. This is especially important if you have no close family or friends. You may also appoint a power of attorney to enforce your wishes.

Physician Orders for Life-Saving Treatment (POLST)

This is a simpler form of the advance directive designed to let your desires be known to the 911 medical personnel who respond to a call from your home. The POLST form is typically posted in a visible

COMMON QUESTIONS ABOUT END-OF-LIFE ISSUES

Q: *What is comfort care? Does this mean I will not receive medications or treatment?*

A: Choosing comfort care means that you do not want aggressive measures such as intubation or chest compressions. However, it does not mean that all treatment will be withheld. Your health-care providers will do everything possible to make sure you are comfortable in your final hours or days of life. You will be provided with medication and treatment that ensures you are not suffering and will not be abandoned by your doctor, nurse, or respiratory therapist.

Q: *What is hospice care? How do I know if this is the right choice for me?*

A: Hospice care focuses on comfort and support rather than treatment for those who are terminally ill. Their team of doctors, nurses, family members, and volunteers provides relief of symptoms as well as emotional and spiritual support. Hospice is reserved for those with a limited life expectancy (typically six months or less) and allows them to spend their remaining months at home.

Q: *What is a durable power of attorney of health care? Do I need one if I have an advance directive or living will?*

A: A durable power of attorney for health care (DPAHC) is a legal directive that allows you to appoint someone as your health-care agent to make decisions for your medical care in the event that you cannot. Choose your agent carefully. Make sure he or she is someone you trust, who knows you well, and who lives nearby. It is a good idea to also choose an alternate in case your primary health-care agent is unavailable.

It is a good idea to appoint a DPAHC even if you have a living will or advance directive. Your DPAHC can help to ensure that your wishes are carried out in the event that your immediate family is unable or unwilling to do so.

Q: *What is a living will?*

A: A living will is simply another name for an advance directive.

place such as on your refrigerator and is the only way for emergency personnel to know your advance directives. Emergency personnel are required to perform resuscitation, including intubation and chest compressions, unless the form is present or your family is available to let your wishes be known. This form is for emergency personnel only and does not replace the advance directive used by the hospital.

CHAPTER 8

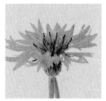

Breathing More Effectively: ("Huff and Puff and Blow the House Down")

Those with COPD may not breathe effectively for several reasons. Panic due to breathlessness may cause you to breathe more quickly and shallowly, making it difficult for your lungs to exchange oxygen and carbon dioxide and tiring your accessory breathing muscles. Air trapping or bronchospasm may make it difficult to take a deep breath. Too much mucus trapped in the airways can cause shortness of breath or impaired gas exchange.

Learning new ways to breathe can help control your shortness of breath, decrease your respiratory rate, improve the exchange of oxygen and carbon dioxide, as well as retrain your body to use your diaphragm for breathing rather than the less-effective accessory breathing muscles.

Pursed-Lip Breathing

Pursed-lip breathing helps to maintain positive pressure in your lungs when you exhale. This positive pressure not only holds floppy airways open, thereby allowing you to exhale stale air that may be trapped, but it also increases the amount of air you can take into your lungs. This allows for better gas exchange, increasing your oxygen and decreasing your carbon dioxide levels. It also helps you focus on your breathing, allowing you to control your shortness of breath and to relax. It is especially helpful for shortness of breath that occurs as a result of exertion or panic.

Technique

1. Breathe in slowly through your nose for a count of two and concentrate on relaxing. You may want to close your eyes and visualize a relaxing scene.

2. Purse your lips as if you were going to whistle.

3. Breathe out gently and slowly through pursed lips for a count of four. Let the air escape through your pursed lips naturally. Do not force the air from your lungs.

4. Keep doing pursed-lip breathing until you are no longer short of breath. Try to relax as you practice pursed-lip breathing.

Abdominal Breathing

Abdominal breathing is another way to help you control your breathing and strengthen your diaphragm. It also helps to expand your lungs so that they can take in more air. This process will not only decrease your respiratory rate but also improve the exchange of oxygen and carbon dioxide.

Technique

1. Sit in a comfortable chair, using good posture.

2. Relax your shoulders.

3. Put one hand on your stomach. As you inhale through your nose, make your stomach push against your hand.

4. Suck in your stomach muscles and exhale through pursed lips. You should feel your stomach move inward.

5. Repeat for three to four breaths. Then rest for two minutes.

6. Repeat this exercise many times a day.

The Walking-Breath Exercise

The walking-breath exercise can be practiced in your home or while on your daily walk. With your eyes open, begin to walk while paying attention to your breathing. Count how many steps you take as you inhale and how many steps you take as you exhale. Try to time the beginning of each inhalation and each exhalation with the time your foot hits the ground. For instance, if you take four steps during each inhalation and four with each exhalation, count *in* 1...2...3...4 and then count *out* 1...2...3...4. Use abdominal breathing and pursed-lip breathing if necessary. Soon you will develop a soothing rhythm that will help to alleviate anxiety and panic.

Control Your Cough

Uncontrolled coughing or difficulty in coughing up mucus can cause shortness of breath. Learning to control your cough will help. Sit in a comfortable chair and perform the following exercise:

1. Take three breaths using pursed lips before trying to cough. Concentrate on relaxing. Close your eyes and visualize a peaceful scene.

2. Sit up and lean your head slightly forward.

3. Take a slow, deep breath through your nose and make sure your muscles are relaxed.

4. Cough once gently (to loosen mucus), using your stomach muscles.

5. Cough a second time (to move mucus forward). Use your stomach muscles with each cough.

6. Wait a few seconds.

7. Sniff gently to inhale. (If you take a big breath, it may push the mucus back into the lungs, making you cough again).

8. Relax.

Repeat steps 3 through 7 if you still feel the need to cough. This exercise is called controlled coughing. It works best when the mucus in your lungs has been thinned by the consumption of lots of fluids. (Drink eight to ten glasses of water every day, if allowed.) Do controlled coughing with small, short coughs. Avoid large blasts of air.

Airway Clearance

Airway clearance is the removal of excess mucus from the lungs through coughing. Thick or large amounts of mucus in the lungs not only make it difficult to breathe but also cause mucus plugging. Dried or retained mucus in the lungs plug up the smaller airways, causing shortness of breath and air trapping.

There are several simple devices such as the Flutter and the Acapella that are available to help loosen mucus and improve your ability to move secretions from your lungs. Similar to the effects of pursed-lip breathing, a valve in these devices creates positive pressure in the lungs in addition to a vibration that can be felt in the chest, both of which work together to loosen mucus. Both of these devices work best if used after a bronchodilator treatment and if you are well hydrated.

Airway-clearance devices require a prescription from your doctor and are available from many providers of home oxygen and respiratory services. Most insurance companies will cover these devices with proper documentation from your health-care provider.

Technique

Each device comes with specific instructions for its use; however, as a general rule you should observe the following procedure.

- Sit in a comfortable chair, in an upright position.
- Inhale until your lungs are three-quarters full.
- Hold your breath for two to three seconds.
- Exhale through the device. Try not to cough.

Do this exercise for five to ten breaths, and then use a controlled cough to expel secretions.

The Vest

The Vest is an airway clearance device designed to be placed around your chest. It creates vibrations that help to loosen secretions in the smaller airways and move them to the larger airways where they can be more easily expelled. The Vest may be used for ten to twenty minutes several times a day depending on your needs and your doctor's recommendation. It is available by prescription only and can be obtained from home oxygen companies and on the Internet. This device is typically covered by medical insurance with proper documentation from your health-care provider.

Relaxation Techniques

The use of relaxation techniques such as deep breathing, visualization, meditation, or yoga can be used to counteract the negative effects of stress. Practiced regularly, relaxation techniques not only reduce levels of everyday stress but also may help to decrease anxiety and allow you to cope more effectively with episodes of shortness of breath.

When experiencing stress, whether it is mental or physical, the body releases chemicals that trigger the "flight-or-fight" response. When the stress response is activated over a long period of time, the effects of these chemicals wear down the body.

These chemicals, called catecholamines, cause your heart to beat faster and your blood pressure to increase. Your breathing becomes rapid and your muscles tense. Prolonged or constant stress can cause hypertension, headaches, fatigue, insomnia, and a weakened immune system.

How to Get Started

A relaxation routine must be done on a regular basis in order to fully reap the benefits. Staying in practice will allow you to use your relaxation technique easily when you feel anxious or short of breath. Set aside a time once or twice a day when you are not sleepy or likely to be interrupted. There are many relaxation techniques to choose from, so pick one that appeals to you and stick to it. You will be amazed at how much better you feel.

A Simple Relaxation Technique

- Sit in a comfortable chair and close your eyes.
- Concentrate on relaxing your muscles. Start at your toes and work your way upward.
- Breathe naturally through your nose. After you have relaxed all the muscles in your body, take some slow, deep breaths. Breathe in through your nose and out through your mouth.
- Sit quietly for five to ten minutes when you are done.
- Practice this technique once or twice daily for at least twenty minutes.

Visualization Techniques

Visualization techniques are helpful during periods of stress, anxiety, or shortness of breath. By visualizing a pleasant scene or memory, you take the focus off your breathing and help your body relax.

Start by closing your eyes and taking some slow, deep breaths. Imagine a place or time where you felt relaxed and at peace. Try using all your senses when visualizing your special place. Hear the sounds, inhale the smells, and feel the positive emotions associated with this place. Let the vision take you away from the immediate stress of your life and soothe your mind, body, and soul.

CHAPTER 9

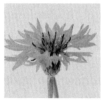

Exercise for Life

Like many people, Mary was not excited about the prospect of starting a daily exercise routine.

> "My walk around the neighborhood is the best part of my day. But I'll tell you, when my doctor first suggested I start walking for exercise, I thought he was nuts. Probably told him so, too.
>
> "But I decided to give it a try. I started out slow.... It took a month before I was even able to get out of the house. Now, here I am, a year later, walking a mile a day and feeling better than I have in years."

After smoking cessation, exercise is the most important thing you can do to improve your quality of life. Participating in a regular exercise routine will allow you to do the things you enjoy with less shortness of breath and greater energy.

Regular exercise not only makes you feel better but it also makes your heart and lungs work better by using oxygen more efficiently, improving circulation, and decreasing blood pressure. It also improves your ability to clear secretions, strengthens your bones, and improves your sleep.

Exercising regularly is an important part of helping yourself gain control of your disease in addition to making you feel better.

Muscles that are not used and are out of shape increase the feeling of breathlessness. Inactivity leads to further muscle loss and over time will actually increase your shortness of breath.

Toned muscles use less oxygen, thereby decreasing your body's overall need for oxygen. The oxygen you do have is put to better use, leaving you more energy to breathe. Many people report that they eat better, sleep better, and breathe better after starting a regular exercise routine.

There are three types of exercise that are particularly important for those with COPD. Aerobic exercise helps improve heart and lung function so that over time it is easier to breathe. Stretching improves flexibility, making it easier to do the things you enjoy, and upper-extremity function builds the strength needed to use the accessory breathing muscles. Before starting any exercise program, it is important to check with your health-care provider. He or she knows your condition and can recommend a regime that will work best for you. (See Figure 9.1 for ideas.)

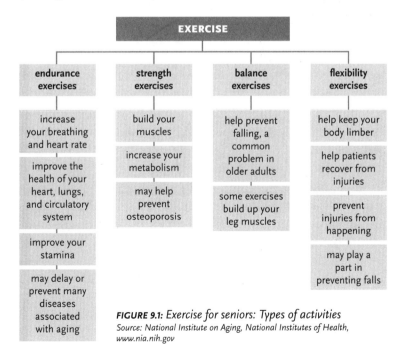

FIGURE 9.1: *Exercise for seniors: Types of activities*
Source: National Institute on Aging, National Institutes of Health, www.nia.nih.gov

Aerobic Exercise

Aerobic exercise such as walking, swimming, or dancing builds endurance. Before you begin an aerobic exercise program, set a realistic goal. Start slowly, exercising at a comfortable pace for a few minutes or longer, twice a day. Aim to work up to twenty minutes for each walk, increasing your time by one or two minutes each session.

Walking is probably one of the safest and easiest ways to exercise. Walk at a comfortable pace and stop short of exhaustion or any feelings of weakness. Remember that mild shortness of breath is not harmful to your heart or lungs. Use pursed-lip breathing if necessary. Walking one or more miles a day is a realistic goal, even if you have severely impaired lungs.

As you increase your walking distance, you will probably find that any shortness of breath comes later and later during exercise. Some people use distractions such as walking with friends or listening to music to desensitize themselves to the discomfort of shortness of breath. Leaning forward while walking may also improve breathing.

Walk outdoors on nice days and in shopping malls in poor weather. Many shopping malls have distances marked off for walkers and offer the added advantage of restrooms at convenient locations. If you do not live near a mall or other good place to walk, you can benefit from other forms of exercise, such as using a treadmill or stationary bike. Many community programs, like chair aerobics, are available. Check at your local senior center or Better Breathers Club for available exercise programs.

Don't push yourself too hard. Doing too much and becoming extremely short of breath or unable to get out of bed the next day is discouraging as well as harmful. Be sure to use your oxygen if prescribed and use pursed-lip breathing while exercising. These measures will decrease your feeling of breathlessness while ensuring your muscles have a plentiful supply of oxygen.

When done regularly, exercise becomes a pleasure instead of a chore. Over time, you may find yourself looking forward to your walk or your dance class. Small changes, such as losing five pounds or sleeping better, will help to keep you motivated and encourage you to continue. If you have difficulty sticking to a routine, recruit your spouse or a friend to exercise with you. It is harder to make excuses to someone else than to yourself.

Flexibility

Whether swimming, walking, or riding a stationary bike, it is important to stretch your muscles before you begin. This stretching will not only help to prevent injuries but also will keep your muscles flexible, making it easier for you to do daily activities such as bathing or putting away your groceries.

For the more adventurous, yoga or tai chi are both great ways to increase flexibility as well as improve mobility. Both disciplines focus on relaxation and better breathing and include training of the mind as well as the body. These techniques may help you to better control your breathing, decrease panic and anxiety, and help you to notice the early symptoms of a flare-up, all of which will help to prevent unwanted ER visits or hospitalizations.

Upper-Extremity Training

Many people with COPD use their shoulder muscles to help them breathe. These muscles become tired and make it difficult to complete tasks that require your arms to be raised up, such as washing your hair or putting dishes into a cupboard. Strengthening these muscles can make both these tasks and breathing easier to do. There are many ways to strengthen these muscles, including using resistance machines and free weights. Most health clubs now offer programs for seniors and provide assistance to those interested in increasing their strength. If you prefer to exercise at home, the use of dumbbells, or even a simple broomstick, can strengthen the upper body, including the accessory breathing muscles.

Sample Exercises

The exercises presented below can be done while sitting upright in bed or in a comfortable straight-backed chair, with your feet flat on the floor. Take an old plastic or wooden broomstick and place it across your knees.

Exercise 1: Grasp the broomstick with your palms facing upward. Raise the broomstick upward, to your chin, extend it out in front of you, and then bring it back to your lap. Repeat five times.

Exercise 2: Without changing your grip on the broomstick, raise the broomstick upward to your chin and extend your arms out in front of you. With your arms extended, raise the broomstick up over your head and then back down and into your lap. Repeat five times.

Exercise 3: With palms still facing upward, bring the broomstick up over your head and rotate the broomstick from left to right, then back down into your lap. Repeat five times.

As you become stronger, you will be able to do more sets of five, or you may want to replace your broomstick with hand weights.

Yoga/Tai Chi

The disciplines of yoga and tai chi are excellent for those with COPD because they focus on relaxation and breathing techniques. They also help keep the body limber through stretching exercises. Limber muscles help keep you flexible and improve mobility. These programs include training the mind as well as the body, and this increased awareness of the mind/body connection may help you control your breathing, decrease feelings of panic and anxiety, as well as allow for better identification of symptoms of a flare-up, preventing unwanted emergency room visits or hospitalizations.

Things to Avoid

No matter which exercise method or routine you choose, there are some things you should avoid doing, such as:

- exercises that require heavy lifting or pushing, such as squats or bench presses
- activities such as shoveling, mowing, or raking

- exercises that require pushing your body against a stationary object, such as push-ups
- exercising outdoors when it is too hot, too cold, humid, or when the air quality is poor
- climbing steep hills

Pulmonary Rehabilitation Programs

Pulmonary rehabilitation programs are an excellent resource for those with COPD who would like to build strength and increase flexibility, endurance, and upper-body strength. Not only do these programs provide valuable information about the disease process, their formal program format can help you achieve your exercise goals in a supervised and monitored environment. Talk with your health-care provider or staff members at your local hospital about pulmonary rehabilitation programs in your area.

CHAPTER 10

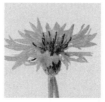

Nutrition: Food Is Energy—Energy Is Life

Proper nutrition is the cornerstone to good health. Food provides your body with the energy it needs to function and those with COPD require even more energy than those with healthy lungs...as much as ten times more.

People with healthy lungs take breathing for granted. However, when your lungs become damaged or diseased, it takes more work to obtain the oxygen your body needs. This increased work and energy can cause tiredness, weight loss, depression, and other negative factors.

Because having lung disease requires more work to breathe, good nutrition is important to replenish the extra energy used in the process. A well-nourished body is better equipped to fight infection. In addition, eating sensibly will give you the energy to accomplish the goals you have set.

Choosing the Right Foods

Food becomes fuel for your body by interacting with oxygen. Low oxygen levels can lead to poor nutrition despite an adequate caloric intake. In addition, choosing the wrong foods may lead to an increase in carbon dioxide levels because carbon dioxide is a waste product of *metabolism* (the conversion of food to energy). Carbon dioxide is carried from your cells in the blood to your lungs and it is removed through the breathing process. Avoid choosing foods that produce a lot of carbon dioxide when metabolized, such as soda pop, candy, and pastries, which consist mainly of sugar (simple carbohydrates) and have little nutritional value. Eating a lot of simple carbohydrates can lead to headache, fatigue, and shortness of breath, especially if you already have higher-than-normal carbon-dioxide levels due to air trapping.

The three major nutrients—carbohydrates, protein, and fat— found in the food you eat are metabolized in different ways. Each requires different amounts of oxygen to process, and each type of nutrient produces different amounts of carbon dioxide as waste. What you eat affects how much carbon dioxide your body must eliminate.

Carbohydrates

Carbohydrates give your body energy. Foods high in carbohydrates, such as bread, pasta, and potatoes, are great for marathon runners but are not the best choice for those with COPD. This is because the metabolism of carbohydrates creates a lot of carbon dioxide—more than any other nutrient. This may cause you to breathe deeper and faster in an attempt to get rid of the excess—something you do not want to do if you already have trouble breathing. Choose complex carbohydrates like whole-wheat bread or cereals high in fiber, which metabolize more slowly.

Protein

Protein helps build muscle, blood, and body tissues. Diets high in protein work well for body builders but not for those with COPD. Like carbohydrates, the metabolism of protein can create an increase in carbon dioxide, making you work harder to breathe.

Fat

Fat makes food taste better and is typically restricted on a weight-loss diet, but it is the best source of energy for those with COPD.

The metabolism of fat creates the least amount of carbon dioxide, while providing your body with the most calories per unit, making it easier to boost your caloric intake, especially if you are underweight. Replacing foods higher in carbohydrates with those higher in fat can help to decrease the amount of work you have to put into breathing while keeping your weight at a healthy level.

■ A Word about Cholesterol

Not all foods high in fat are high in bad cholesterol—a relief for those watching their cholesterol levels. Fat that is high in bad cholesterol is called saturated fat, and it typically comes from animal sources such as lard. These fats are easy to spot because they are typically solid at cool temperatures. Polyunsaturated or monounsaturated fats are a healthier choice. They usually come from plant sources such as canola, sunflower, or corn, and they can be used for cooking to boost your fat intake.

Steps to Good Nutritional Health

By following a few healthy steps, such as limiting your salt intake and maintaining a healthy weight, you will be on the road to enjoying better nutritional health. And when your nutritional health improves, so will your COPD symptoms.

Maintain a Healthy Weight

Talk with your health-care provider about what is a healthy weight for you and how many calories you should consume in a day. Being either underweight or overweight can make breathing more difficult. If you are underweight, your body simply does not have the extra energy required to breathe effectively. If you are overweight, your body demands even more oxygen, making it difficult to breathe.

Monitor your weight on a regular basis to help you stay on track. Weighing yourself once or twice a week (unless your health-care provider recommends weighing more often) will alert you to any changes that may be signs of an impending problem. If you are taking diuretics or oral steroids such as prednisone your weight may fluctuate; however, if you notice an unexplained weight gain of two or more pounds in one day or greater than five pounds in a week, it is important that you contact your health-care provider.

■ What If I Am Underweight?

It may be difficult to eat enough calories to efficiently fuel your body. If you are trying to gain weight, choose snacks that are nutrition dense, such as peanut butter, hard-boiled eggs, and tuna fish. There are also many good liquid nutritional supplements that are tasty and provide a lot of calories with the right balance of carbohydrates, fats, and proteins.

Keep Yourself Hydrated

Drinking at least six 8-oz. glasses of water a day (unless your doctor recommends otherwise) will help keep you hydrated and make mucus thinner and easier to cough up. If you don't like to drink plain water, drink six 8-oz glasses of noncaffeinated beverages. You should limit your caffeine intake because it can interfere with some of your medications.

■ Important Facts about Water

Did you know...?

- Two-thirds of Americans are chronically dehydrated.
- The number-one cause of daytime fatigue is a lack of water.
- For many people, the thirst mechanism is so weak that it is often mistaken for hunger.
- A 2 percent drop in the body's water intake can trigger fuzzy short-term memory.
- Chronic dehydration is the root of many serious diseases, including asthma, kidney dysfunction, endocrine and adrenal fatigue, high blood pressure and other heart problems, arthritis, ulcers, pancreatitis, digestive problems, and lower-back pain.
- The mucus that lines the stomach to protect it from stomach acid consists of 98 percent water.

- Drinking five glasses of water daily may decrease the risk of colon cancer by almost 50 percent and decreases the risk of breast cancer by 80 percent.
- A dry mouth is the very last sign of dehydration.
- Every function of the body is monitored and regulated by the flow of water.

Eat a Balanced Diet

Eating a balanced diet consists of selecting a wide variety of foods that are packed with nutrition. Therefore, you must eat a diet that includes meat, dairy products, fruits, vegetables, and bread and cereals. Meat and dairy products contain protein, the building blocks of muscle. Fruits and vegetables are filled with vitamins and minerals. Breads and cereals contain fiber, which helps to maintain a healthy digestive system, and carbohydrates, which provide energy to your entire body.

The FDA's Daily Food Pyramid suggests consuming the following portions:

- 3–5 servings of fresh or steamed vegetables a day. A serving size is ½ cup. Keep in mind that canned vegetables contain a lot of sodium.
- 2–4 servings of fresh fruit a day. A serving size is a medium-size apple, banana, peach, etc., or ½ cup of canned fruit. Be aware that canned fruit typically contains a lot of sugar.
- 6–11 servings of bread, cereal, rice, or pasta. A serving size is 1 slice of bread, ½ cup of cereal, pasta, or rice.
- 2–3 servings of meat. A serving size is 1 oz. Lean meat and poultry should be your number-one choice.
- 2–3 servings of milk, yogurt, or cheese. A serving is 1 cup of milk or yogurt or 1½ ounces of sliced cheese.
- Fats, sweets, and alcohol should be used sparingly.

Keep in mind that different people have different needs. For example, people on diuretics may need to increase their potassium intake by eating foods such as bananas, oranges, potatoes, tomatoes, or asparagus. Your health-care provider can help you develop a nutrition plan tailored to your individual needs.

Watch Your Salt Intake

Too much salt causes the body to retain water, which makes it harder to breathe. The recommended daily intake of salt (sodium) is less than 2,000 mg. Some tricks to reducing your salt intake include the following:

- Remove the saltshaker from your table.
- Use herbs and spices rather than salt.
- Don't add salt when you are cooking.
- Read food labels.
- Use a salt substitute.

Avoid Overeating

Avoid eating too much or eating foods that cause bloating. A full stomach not only makes you feel uncomfortable, but it also puts pressure on your diaphragm, making it more difficult for you to breathe. If you are typically getting too full at meals, try breaking them up. For example, if you are eating three big meals a day, break them down into six smaller ones.

If gas or bloating is making you uncomfortable, avoid the following foods:

- carbonated drinks
- apples, broccoli, Brussels sprouts, cabbage, corn, cucumbers, beans, melons, onions, and peppers
- deep-fried foods

Healthy Habits

Helen, age fifty-six, became so short of breath that she dreaded mealtimes: "I got short of breath, so I couldn't eat. I finally decided to do something about it. Now I sit at my kitchen table for all meals. I always wear my oxygen, and now instead of gulping my food I take smaller bites and chew slowly."

Why does this work? Sitting at the table to eat encourages good posture. Good posture allows the diaphragm to work properly. Wearing oxygen provides the body with enough to contribute to metabolism and energy. Taking small bites and chewing slowly helps with digestion and prevents you from overeating.

Others have reported that choosing foods that are easy to prepare and easy to chew decreases their shortness of breath. Drink at the end of the meal rather than at the beginning, in order to leave plenty of room for your food. And always, always use pursed-lip breathing.

If you are having difficulty with preparing meals, don't be afraid to ask a family member to help, or check with your local Meals on Wheels organization or senior center. Don't look at this option as "needing help." You are simply maximizing your energy.

More Healthy Meal Tips

- Rest before eating.
- Avoid lying down after meals.
- Eat your main meal early if you are too tired to eat later in the day.
- Add margarine, mayonnaise, or other sources of fat to bread and vegetables. If you are watching your cholesterol level, use polyunsaturated fats, oils, and margarine.
- Ask for help with grocery shopping and/or cooking from friends or family members.
- Limit fluids at meals if they make you feel too full to eat.
- Use artificially sweetened jams, jellies, and hard candies and avoid "empty" carbohydrates such as candy and sugar.
- Eat lots of fresh fruits and vegetables. Although they contain carbohydrates, they also contain the important nutrients your body needs.

Supplements

There are a variety of nutritional supplements that may be beneficial for those with COPD.

Vitamin C (Ascorbic Acid): Vitamin C is an essential vitamin that has antioxidant properties. It helps to build collagen and connective tissue, which makes it important for healing. Vitamin C is found in citrus fruits and vegetables, such as red and green peppers, tomatoes, potatoes, and spinach or collard greens.

Vitamin E: Vitamin E also has antioxidant properties and is essential for the healing of wounds. It also helps to prevent plaque buildup, maintains a healthy nervous system, and acts as an anti-inflammatory. Vitamin E can be found in wheat germ oil, tomato products, sunflower seed oil and kernels, almonds, and spinach.

Niacin: Niacin is a B vitamin that is responsible for the production of energy and is involved in the repair of tissues. It can lower cholesterol and decrease the risk of heart disease and stroke. Niacin is found in meat, poultry, fish, and beans.

Zinc: Zinc is an essential mineral that acts as an anti-inflammatory, helps to balance blood sugar, builds teeth and bones, and helps maintain the immune system. Zinc is found in oysters, eggs, liver and red meat, fish, poultry, black-eyed peas, and whole grains.

Calcium: Calcium is an essential mineral that builds the teeth and bones, as well as regulates the heart rhythm. Calcium is especially important if you are taking steroids, because they cause bone to break down. Calcium is found in dairy products, fish, shellfish, and raw tofu.

Potassium: Potassium is an essential mineral as well as one of the three major electrolytes in the body. It helps regulate blood pressure and maintain the acid/base balance, the function of the muscles and nerves, the production of energy, and kidney function. Potassium is found in avocados, lima beans, potatoes, tomatoes, apricots, bananas, chicken, and fish. Those on heart medications should consult their health-care provider before taking potassium supplements.

CHAPTER 11

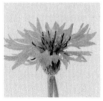

Setting Your Goals for Change

Imagine sitting on your couch one cold winter day and seeing a travel commercial for Florida showing white beaches, blue surf, and lots of sunshine. That looks great, you think. Nice and warm! You decide Florida is the place to be.

Do you immediately jump in your car and take off? Of course not. At the very least you would consult a road map or AAA, talk it over with friends or family, and review guidebooks to get the most out of your experience.

When planning a trip, you need to determine not only where you are going but also how you are going to get there. The same is true of your journey to better living. To accomplish your goals, you must create a realistic plan. You may need help from professionals, such as your doctor or respiratory therapist, and support from good friends or family.

You've been working hard in previous chapters. You've learned a lot about your disease, your triggers, and how to breathe more efficiently. You have the tools you need to succeed. Let's put these tools to good use and create your plan for change.

Think back to the beginning of this book. Remember the three things you listed that you would like to do again. Now is the time to decide if these three things are realistic or if they need to be modified. For example, you may not be able to swim six miles anymore, but you could join the YMCA and take a water aerobics class. There are many different ways to do what you enjoy. It just takes a little thought and determination. Once you have three realistic goals in mind, you are ready for the next step.

Plan Your Trip for Better Living

You've decided on a goal. Now you need to plan how you are going to accomplish this goal. It won't happen overnight. A step-by-step plan is crucial to achieving your goal. Decide now if your original goals are realistic or require modification. Once you have some realistic goals in mind, you are ready for the next step.

When Are You Leaving? When Do You Want to Arrive? Having a start date is important. It need not be today. It might be tomorrow or next week. Give yourself enough plenty of time to plan and prepare. If you start before you have everything in order, you may be setting yourself up for failure.

Your completion date is equally important. It shows that you are committed to your plan and provides motivation.

Who Is Coming Along for the Ride? There is no need to go it alone. Friends, family, support groups, and medical professionals are an important part of your plan. Who can you count on for support?

How Are You Going to Get There? Do you have the tools you need to succeed? Do you have your support systems in place? Make sure you are prepared in order to succeed.

Pulmonary Rehabilitation

Enrolling in a formal pulmonary rehabilitation program may be the best way for you to achieve your goals. A formal program gives you the opportunity to work with a team of experts dedicated to helping you succeed. This team may include physicians, respiratory therapists, nurses, dieticians, and social workers so that a wide range of concerns or issues may be addressed.

Is Pulmonary Rehabilitation Right for You?

Participation in a pulmonary rehabilitation program is work, and just like any other activity it requires the time and energy necessary to do the work involved. You must also be committed—both to the program and to feeling better.

People with moderate COPD (FEV$_1$ > 60 percent predicted) seem to reap the most benefit from a formal program. Those without symptoms or with end-stage disease are not usually recommended for the program. Many programs require you to be a nonsmoker or at least be attempting to quit, and most programs can help you if you are having difficulty. It is also important to have a friend or family member who is supportive of your efforts in the program. To be considered for pulmonary rehabilitation, your health-care provider must refer you to the program, so talk to your provider if pulmonary rehab interests you.

What Happens Next?

You will meet with a member of the pulmonary rehabilitation team for an assessment. This assessment will determine if you meet the requirements to enroll. If you do—congratulations—you are on your way to better health!

Most programs meet twice a week for several months. Early on, tests will be conducted to help you set realistic, measurable goals based on your individual needs and abilities. You will also receive education about your disease, your medications, and your equipment—all in a supportive environment.

What Are the Benefits?

George Sanders started smoking at age thirteen. By the time he was forty, he was smoking over two packs a day. He began to notice some mild shortness of breath when climbing the steps in and out of the school bus he drove for a living, but he wrote it off to being out of shape.

As the years went on, George experienced more episodes of breathlessness, especially when climbing stairs, so he began to decrease his activity level as much as possible. As a result, he gained fifty pounds over a period of ten years.

He began coughing up thick mucus every morning, which he called just a "smoker's cough." Ignoring his wife's concerns over his health, he continued to smoke, and the only exercise he got was while at work, which wasn't much. George really felt like he was fine; after all, he was almost age fifty-five, and as far as he was concerned, his symptoms were just a normal part of getting older. He went to his doctor, who diagnosed him with COPD, gave him an inhaler, and told him to come back if his symptoms worsened. Although his doctor recommended further testing, George did not follow through because he felt that his doctor was overreacting.

On the morning of his fifty-fifth birthday, George woke up with what he described as a "chest cold." He stayed home from work for three days, taking over-the-counter cold remedies; painfully coughing up thick, yellow-green sputum; and telling his concerned wife that he was not going to make an appointment with his doctor no matter how much she nagged, so just leave him alone. She did so, until she found him unconscious in his recliner, struggling to breathe. Then she called 911.

When the paramedics arrived, they found his oxygen levels to be dangerously low and his heart rate just as dangerously high. They quickly pulled him to the floor, placed a tube in his throat, and began to breathe for him using high levels of oxygen. They hooked him up to a monitor, started an IV, and then loaded him into the ambulance in a race to the hospital.

His heart stopped the minute he went through the emergency room doors. His frantic wife was ushered out of the room while medical personnel rushed to save his life. After several minutes of chest compressions and medications designed to jump-start George's heart, it began to beat on its own again.

Once he was stabilized, George was moved to the critical care unit, where doctors, nurses, respiratory therapists, and other health-care professionals worked around the clock to treat the pneumonia that had overwhelmed his body. They administered antibiotics, steroids, and bronchodilators. He had a tube down his throat and another down his nose, and he was hooked up to monitors, IV pumps, and a ventilator for over a week. His pneumonia was so bad that at one point early on, his doctor wasn't sure he would survive.

"I was so angry with him, " his wife, Jeannine, says. "Every time I tried to talk to George about losing weight or quitting smoking, he would just come unglued. I only brought it up because I love him and wanted to have him around for a good long time, but he always took it as some kind of threat. When he kept accusing me of being a nag, I just gave up talking about it. I felt like if he really loved me and valued our relationship, he would have gotten some exercise and at least *cut back* on his smoking so I wouldn't be sitting here right now by his bedside, praying to God that my husband of thirty-five years doesn't die."

Thankfully, George survived his ordeal and was moved to the general medical floor. After two weeks, he was finally well enough to leave the hospital and go home.

"That experience changed my life," George now says. "I can't say I saw a bright, white light or any of my deceased relatives, but it did make me realize how precious life really is. I mean, my God, I haven't even reached retirement age and my life was almost over, mainly because of what I did to it. Things will never be the same again—in good ways and in bad. I have permanent damage to my lungs from my bout with the pneumonia that almost killed me. I tire out more easily now and still have episodes of shortness of breath, but the minute I got home from the hospital I vowed to take control of my disease and my life."

George enrolled in a twelve-week pulmonary rehabilitation program offered at the same hospital where he almost lost his life. As you can see from George's story, participating in a pulmonary rehab program can improve your quality of life. Other graduates of pulmonary rehab programs describe having:

- increased physical endurance
- increased muscle strength
- increased energy

- improved breathing with less shortness of breath
- a better understanding of their disease
- better nutrition
- less anxiety and panic
- improved intimacy with their partner
- more self-confidence

With all of the potential benefits that can come from entering a pulmonary rehab program, it is a wise choice for improving your quality of life.

CHAPTER 12

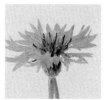

Tips and Tricks
for Daily Living

When you wake up in the morning, do you feel excited about the day ahead or do you dread getting up and trying to accomplish your activities of daily living such as grooming, cleaning, or fixing meals? People with healthy lungs take these basic tasks for granted, never realizing how difficult these simple things can be for someone with COPD. But do not despair. Learning to accomplish these tasks more efficiently will help you to do more with less discomfort from shortness of breath and fatigue. Try some of the ideas in this chapter and, as always, take your breathing medication, wear your oxygen, and used pursed-lip breathing when doing your daily chores to maximize your energy and decrease your feelings of breathlessness.

In the Bedroom

Just getting out of bed and getting dressed for the day can be quite an ordeal if you have COPD. Doing as much as possible while sitting conserves energy. Laying your clothes out the day before on a dresser top or nightstand will eliminate any bending or reaching you have to do first thing in the morning. Get dressed while sitting on your bed or in a straight-backed chair and make sure your shoes are close by. If bending causes you to become short of breath, get a long-handled shoehorn to help you put them on and be sure to buy shoes that are easy to slip on. The more time you spend tying or fastening your shoes, the more short of breath you may become.

Make sure your entire bedroom is user-friendly. Organize your clothes so that they are easy to reach and avoid using the bottom drawers of your dresser if possible. Instead, hang these clothes up in your closet or wardrobe and make sure you choose clothing that is easy to fasten or that slips easily over your head. Avoid tight clothing because it will make breathing more difficult.

Get rid of excess quilts, comforters, or pillows and replace them with linen that is lightweight so that your bed is easier to make. If you get cold at night, use an electric blanket rather than a heavy down-filled quilt. Don't waste energy when making your bed because you'll need that energy later in the day.

Bathing/Showering

Grooming can be a challenge if you have COPD, but some simple modifications can make it easier. For example, getting into and out of a bathtub can be difficult as well as dangerous. If possible, have your bathtub converted into a walk-in shower stall. If this cannot be done, prevent slips with rugs or carpeting and place anti-slip decals in the bathtub itself. Avoid lying down in the bathtub as if may be difficult to get up—especially if you become short of breath. Install a shower wand that fits on the tub spout and consider getting a bath bench. This will allow you to sit while bathing, conserving your energy and decreasing your degree of shortness of breath.

Whether you have a bathtub or shower stall, installing grab bars can make it easier for you to get in and out as well as help to prevent falls. Make sure all of your soaps and shampoos are handy. Shower organizers are inexpensive and available almost anywhere and can be mounted within arm's reach.

Grooming

Once again, sitting is best, so apply your makeup, do your hair, and/or shave while sitting down. If the mirror in your bathroom is too high, have one mounted lower or use a makeup mirror at your kitchen table. Try to avoid aerosol grooming products or those that have strong fragrances, because they may irritate your lungs.

In the Kitchen

Preparing and eating meals should be a pleasure not a chore. A little reorganization can go a long way toward making your meals enjoyable again.

Store utensils, plates, cups, and other frequently used items in cupboards that are within easy reach and use electric appliances such as can openers to conserve energy. The addition of a microwave oven allows you to not only prepare meals with less work but also to warm up extra food you have prepared on a good day. Making extra and freezing in simple meal portions saves time and precious energy. These meals are great to warm up when you are having a bad day.

Do as much meal preparation as you can while sitting at your kitchen table. Grating, peeling, chopping, and slicing can easily be done while sitting down, using a cutting board on the tabletop.

Housework

When cleaning, remember you are not running the one hundred–yard dash. With a little planning, you will find that your housework does not have to be overwhelming or exhausting. Divide your tasks into manageable blocks. Perhaps you can clean the bathroom on Saturdays instead of every day. All of your chores do not need to be done in one day. And if you can't get to everything—so what, it'll still be there tomorrow. Stop and rest frequently. If you overdo it one day, it will be even harder to do more the next.

You may want to purchase a little pushcart to help carry your cleaning products or to help carry those things you pick up around the house. And speaking of cleaning products, be careful when using them because the fumes may irritate your lungs. Wear a mask if necessary while using these products, as well as while dusting, to prevent dust particles from causing bronchospasm and shortness of breath.

Out and About

Don't let COPD hold you prisoner in your own home. There is no reason to feel trapped. As long as you plan ahead, you can get out and run errands or do the things you enjoy. If you use oxygen, be sure to bring enough so that you don't run out and have to interrupt your plans.

You may want to consider getting a handicap permit. These permits are available at the DMV with proper documentation from your health-care provider. By parking closer to the building, you can save your energy for inside the store rather than wasting it walking across a parking lot.

Remember not to shop during peak hours or on weekends. A crowded store makes shopping more difficult. Choose grocery stores with employees who will help with your groceries. Another energy saver to consider is shopping through mail order or the Internet and be sure to use pharmacies that offer home delivery.

Home Safety

According to the Home Safety Council, slips and falls are the leading cause of death from home injuries. Approximately 5.1 million people over the age of sixty-five are injured from falls in their home, and one-third of these injuries result in death. Home safety is particularly important for those with COPD. Oral steroids can cause bones to become brittle and easier to break if a fall occurs. Home medical equipment may create obstacles, causing you to trip or fall over electrical cords or oxygen tubing. Give your home a safety checkup using the following information as a guide:

Outside

- Make sure steps and walkways are in good repair. Check for cracks in the concrete, abrupt edges, and loose or broken boards.

- Ensure that porch railings are easy to use and are not loose or wobbly.

- Outside lights should provide enough light for you to easily see your porch, walkway, and yard.

Living Room/Den

- Doorways should be wide enough to accommodate wheelchairs, walkers, and other medical equipment.

- Keep pathways through your home clear of clutter or debris.

- Electric and phone cords should not run under rugs, carpet, or across open areas.

- Consider purchasing a cordless phone that can be placed in your pocket or walker basket, allowing you phone access throughout your home.

- Test your smoke detectors monthly.

- Make sure light switches are easy to reach and will light the room before you enter. Make sure you have adequate lighting for every room.

Bathroom

- Purchase raised toilet seats to make getting on and off the toilet easier.

- Put in a nightlight to provide illumination for nighttime bathroom visits.

- Set the hot water heater to below 120° F to prevent scalding.

- Ensure telephone access by installing a phone jack in the bathroom or always bringing your charged cordless phone with you.

Bedroom

- Avoid throw rugs, which can bunch and cause a fall.

- Keep the floor clear of clutter.

Kitchen

- Avoid clutter in the kitchen.
- Have a fire extinguisher handy and know how to use it.

Emergency Response Devices

Emergency response devices such as Life Alert help you to get emergency services in the event that you cannot reach a telephone. When you sign up for this service, you will be provided with a pendant-shaped device that can be worn as a necklace or wristband. This device is connected to a phone line and there is an emergency dispatcher on the other end. The device is wireless so there is no need to add extra equipment or phone lines.

One press of the button activates the auto dialer and connects you with the company's emergency dispatcher by speakerphone. The dispatcher will alert EMS and get them to you quickly.

The pendant is lightweight, easy to use, and waterproof, so there is no need to take it off. Some insurance companies will even reimburse you for the cost of these devices, but even if they do not, it is well worth the expense.

CHAPTER 13

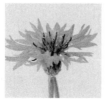

Taking It on the Road: Traveling with COPD

Jane was devastated when she learned she had to wear home oxygen. She and her husband had just bought a new motor home and had planned to travel extensively. But rather than let anything stop her, she did some research and learned that with proper planning, their trip would be quite easy.

Having COPD or using home oxygen does not mean you cannot travel. Advances in home oxygen and respiratory equipment have provided those who like to travel with lightweight, battery-operated devices that make traveling easier than ever.

Portable oxygen concentrators: Recent changes in airline policy have made it possible to bring approved oxygen concentrators on board airplanes. These machines typically weigh less than ten pounds and are battery operated. If you are renting a portable concentrator, be sure to get it a couple of days before you plan to leave to make sure it works properly and always charge the batteries the night before you leave. You may want to bring extra batteries and an electrical adapter with extra plugs, especially if traveling by air, to ensure you will always have power to the machine. The batteries last three to ten hours, depending on the model, and most use oxygen-conserving technology. If you require a continuous flow, be sure to let your provider know so that he or she can find a machine that works well for you.

Portable nebulizers: Small battery-operated nebulizers are now available for travel. These machines easily fit in a bag or large purse and are essential if you need breathing treatments during the day and are traveling. Although they may not be covered by your insurance plan, they are well worth the out-of-pocket expense if you are active or traveling.

Careful planning is essential for those with COPD. Make a checklist based on the following information to ensure your trip goes smoothly.

Where Are You Going?

Be sure to research the city or state that you will be visiting. Places at high or low altitude can affect your breathing. You may need to increase your liter flow if on oxygen especially if visiting an area located at a high altitude. Consult with your health-care provider if you are planning to travel at high or low altitudes.

Poor air quality can cause an exacerbation of COPD. Before you leave, call ahead or check air pollution levels to determine if air quality will be an issue. Also, consider the problem of indoor air pollution. Stay at smoke-free hotels or motels.

If you are on supplemental oxygen, ask your home-oxygen provider it they have a branch in the city you will be visiting. Call your home-oxygen provider or stop by and ask for a provider directory.

Are You Healthy Enough to Travel?

Nothing ruins a vacation faster than ending up in a hospital bed. Schedule a visit with your health-care provider shortly before you plan to leave. He or she may want to prescribe extra medication in case of a flare-up while on the road. Your doctor can also provide you with your home-oxygen prescription as well as with any other medical documents that may be required when you travel.

How Will You Get There?

How you travel can also affect your COPD symptoms. Travel by car, air, or rail all present different challenges to consider.

Automobile/RV

If you will be driving for long periods of time, make sure you are prepared. Bring plenty of water to stay hydrated and be sure to keep your medications handy in your purse or travel bag. Be sure to schedule frequent rest stops to stretch and prevent clots from forming in your legs.

If you are driving through areas with high pollution levels or on crowded highways, keep your windows up and turn on the air conditioner to protect your lungs from irritation. Also, try to avoid driving during peak hours.

If you are on supplemental oxygen, know how many oxygen tanks you need to make the entire trip without running out. It is best to take at least one more tank than you think you will need. Talk with your home-oxygen provider before leaving. He or she can provide you with extra tanks for your trip and may be able to help arrange for a concentrator or other device to be provided at your destination. Check with your home-care provider for options if you use more than 6 lpm. Use the handy chart in Table 10.1 to determine how long your oxygen will last when starting with a full tank.

TABLE 10.1: Oxygen Tank Duration Time

Tank Size	Liter Flow			
	1 lpm*	2 lpm	3 lpm	4 lpm
A	1 hr 10 min	38 min	23 min	17 min
B	2 hr 20 min	1 hr 15 min	45 min	34 min
D	5 hrs	2 hrs 56 min	1 hr 15 min	1 hr
E	9 hrs	5 hrs	3 hrs	2 hrs

* lpm = liters per minute

The use of an oxygen-conserving device may be beneficial. These devices can significantly increase the time your oxygen tank will last. They "conserve" oxygen by giving a "burst" of oxygen on inhalation only, rather than running continuously, as with a common regulator. These devices are available from your home-oxygen provider and require a visit from a respiratory therapist to adjust the settings, as a setting of 2 on the oxygen-conserving device does not equal 2 lpm. Oximetry is used to determine which setting keeps you best oxygenated.

Don't smoke or allow others to smoke while in the car. Store your extra oxygen tanks on the floorboards behind the seats or secure them with the seat belt. It is not good to let tanks roll around in the vehicle.

Air Travel

There are special considerations for those with COPD when flying, especially when using supplemental oxygen. Many airlines now allow certain small portable oxygen concentrators on board the aircraft. Check with the airline when making reservations or visit www.copd-international.com. This website provides in-depth information about airline travel, as well as information about which concentrators are approved for use on each airline's aircraft. Most airlines require a copy of your home-oxygen prescription as well as other medical documentation.

Portable oxygen tanks are typically not allowed on board unless empty and stored in the baggage area. Make arrangements for oxygen while in the airport or during layovers, as airports do not typically provide this service. Your home-oxygen provider can help.

Depending on your condition, you may need an increase in liter flow while in the air. Airplanes fly at an altitude that is higher than you are used to, which can cause low oxygen levels, hyperventilation, bloating, or sinus pressure. Talk with your health-care provider before you leave to ensure a safe flight.

Bus

Most bus lines will provide assistance for those with special needs. Call at least forty-eight hours before you plan to leave and let them know if you use supplemental oxygen or are in a wheelchair. Some bus lines will allow a couple of oxygen tanks on board, as well as extras below in stowage. Call ahead for specific regulations.

Train

As with bus travel, call ahead for information about obtaining help with special needs. Amtrak, for example, requires at least twelve hours prior notice of your plans to travel with portable oxygen. Any device brought on board must be able to go four hours without electricity and must weigh no more than fifty pounds. They may allow two to six portable tanks but you must always call ahead, as regulations may change without notice. As always, bring a copy of your oxygen prescription and any additional medical documentation that may be required.

Cruise Ship

Most cruise lines require four to six weeks prior notice if traveling with special needs or supplemental oxygen. This can be arranged through your travel agent or the cruise line itself. They typically allow oxygen concentrators on board; however, cruise line regulations may vary.

Do You Have Everything You Need?

Make a packing list to be sure you have everything you need, including the following:

- sufficient oxygen
- sufficient medication
- a copy of your oxygen prescription
- required medical documentation
- a list of your medications
- proper electrical adapters, particularly if traveling overseas or to foreign countries
- directory of locations of your home-oxygen provider

What If You Become Sick while Traveling?

If you begin to feel ill while traveling, seek medical assistance from a walk-in clinic, urgent-care center, or emergency room. Do not delay care. Get medical assistance early to prevent a medical emergency while traveling.

CHAPTER 14

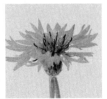

Smoking Cessation: Commit to Quit

The decision to quit smoking is a personal challenge that everyone with COPD must face. Whether you are newly diagnosed or have been living with the disease for years, quitting smoking is the one thing that you can do that will have the most significant impact on your health and will reduce, eliminate, or even reverse the damage done to your lungs.

The Ugly Facts about Cigarettes

Cigarettes contain nicotine, a toxic substance produced by the to-bacco plant that protects it from insects. Although poisonous to the human body at very high levels, it is not what causes damage to the heart, lungs, and other organs. Rather, it is the cigarette itself that leads to COPD, heart disease, and cancer. Cigarettes contain more than four thousand toxic chemicals, such as acetone, formaldehyde, and lead.

Nicotine is the main reason people smoke cigarettes. This is be-cause nicotine is highly addictive—as addictive as heroin or cocaine. A cigarette delivers nicotine to the body the same way a syringe deliv-ers heroin, but much more quickly. Within ten seconds of your first puff, nicotine hits your brain, stimulating the release of dopamine, a "feel-good" chemical, and norepinephrine, which causes the adrenal glands to secrete adrenaline. This causes your heart rate to increase and your arteries and veins to constrict quickly, leading to an increase in blood pressure that increases your risk for a heart attack or stroke.

Toxic chemicals enter the lungs, causing a defense reaction. The larger airways constrict, mucus production increases, and carbon monoxide replaces oxygen in the blood. Cells become irritated, causing the damage that leads to COPD, and over time cells may mutate leading to cancer or death (see Figure 14.1 on the next page).

Nicotine Addiction

Understanding nicotine addiction is crucial to escaping its grasp. Until fairly recently, smoking cigarettes was accepted, if not encouraged; however, it is now known that smoking is hazardous to your health and to those around you. Smoking has become so socially unacceptable that laws have been passed that ban smoking from the workplace, restaurants, bars, and even casinos.

This movement, while well intended, has done little to address nicotine addiction itself. Instead, people who smoke have been labeled bad, weak, or lacking common sense. This label could not be further from the truth and does little to encourage people to quit.

Most people who use tobacco in any form, whether it be through cigarettes, a pipe, or chew, have a *physical* addiction to nicotine. Nicotine stimulates "feel-good" chemicals in the brain called dopamine and serotonin. As nicotine use increases, the body depends on receiving a certain level of it to feel normal.

When nicotine levels decrease, the body has a negative reaction to its removal called withdrawal. Classic symptoms of physical withdrawal from nicotine include:

- tingling in the hands and feet
- sweating
- stomach problems such as nausea, cramping, or constipation

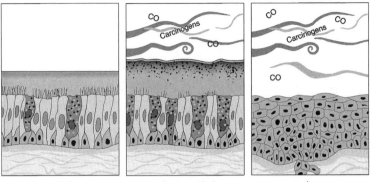

normal bronchial epithelium   a smoker's epithelium   carcinoma

FIGURE 14.1: *The effects of smoking. This three-part image illustrates the effects of smoking on the epithelial cells of the bronchi. The image on the left shows normal, healthy cells in contrast to the image on the right, in which the cells have become cancerous.*

Immediate Effects of Smoking Include the Following:

- One cigarette immediately raises a person's blood pressure and heart rate and decreases the blood flow to body extremities.
- Brain activity and the nervous system are stimulated for a short while and then the stimulation becomes reduced.
- A smoker may experience dizziness, nausea, watery eyes, and acid in the stomach while or after smoking.
- The appetite and senses, such as taste and smell, are distorted.

Smoking Increases the Risk for:

- respiratory infections such as pneumonia and chronic bronchitis
- emphysema
- heart attacks and coronary disease
- cancers, such as lung, throat, mouth, and cervix
- stomach ulcers
- peripheral vascular diseases

Other Effects of Smoking Include:

- shortness of breath
- persistent coughs
- yellow stains on fingers and teeth
- changes in appearance such as facial wrinkles and "rubber"-like skin
- bad-smelling breath, clothes, hair, home, car, etc.
- decreased sense of taste and smell
- weakened immune systems compared to nonsmokers
- possible impotence in men, and women are less fertile than nonsmokers

Other Dangerous Facts about Smoking Include the Following:

- Smoking during pregnancy can affect the unborn child.
- Secondhand smoking is as dangerous, if not more dangerous, than firsthand smoking.
- Smoking in a room separate from children or others does not necessarily avoid secondhand smoking, because carcinogens can seep into furniture and walls.

- headache
- cold symptoms, such as sore throat and coughing
- weight gain

In addition to the physical symptoms of withdrawal, there may be psychological symptoms as well, such as:

- anger
- boredom
- depression
- fatigue
- insomnia

These symptoms are normal, and they occur for a good reason. That cigarette has been your friend for a long time. It has always been there for you through thick and thin. It is normal to mourn the loss of your friend. You may feel angry or depressed, which are both signs of mourning your loss.

Tobacco use may also be linked to events or habits, making it even more difficult to quit, such as:

- eating and drinking
- coffee
- alcohol
- social situations
- stressful situations

For example, it may be more difficult to resist a cigarette with your morning cup of coffee or after a lunch out with friends. Stress at work or at home may trigger a desire to smoke because the body craves those brain chemicals that temporarily make you feel better.

Preparing to Quit

We have all heard stories about people who just put down that pack of cigarettes and never smoke again. If only it were that easy for all of us. Studies have shown that many smokers are unable to quit without careful planning and strong support. Luckily, there are plenty of tools and resources available for those who choose to quit.

Tools to Help You Quit Smoking

When you make the decision to quit smoking, there are many tools available to assist you in becoming nicotine-free. Your health-care provider can assist in choosing the method best suited for you.

■ Nicotine-Replacement Therapy

Nicotine-replacement therapy is designed to gradually wean your body from nicotine until you are drug-free. Nicotine-replacement therapy is not for everyone, and it does not always adequately address the psychological withdrawal symptoms of smoking cessation. However, when used in combination with other methods, it may increase your odds of remaining smoke-free.

Although patches and gum are now available without a prescription, you should talk with your doctor or other health-care provider before using them. People with heart disease, who are pregnant, or who have other health conditions, should not use these products unless authorized by their physician.

In addition, you should never smoke while using these products. Too much nicotine can cause serious and dangerous side effects.

■ Nicotine Gum

Gums such as Nicorette contain nicotine. When chewed, nicotine is released from the gum and absorbed in the mouth, reducing the physical symptoms of nicotine withdrawal. It is not designed to be chewed continually; rather, it should be chewed slowly until you notice a "tingly" sensation and then tucked between your cheek and gums.

When the "tingle" stops, it should be chewed again and then tucked into another spot in your mouth until all of the nicotine in the gum is released—usually after about thirty minutes of chewing and tucking.

Side effects of nicotine gum include:

- mouth sores

- increase in saliva production
- indigestion
- headache

When chewed too fast or continually, nicotine may be swallowed causing:

- dizziness or lightheadedness
- hiccups
- nausea/vomiting
- insomnia

Be aware that nicotine gum can interfere with some medications prescribed for lung disease. Talk with your doctor before using this product.

■ Nicotine Patch

Nicotine patches such as Nicoderm deliver a steady dose of nicotine through the skin. They are available without a prescription and usually come in three doses:

- 21 mg for those who smoke one or more packs per day
- 14 mg for those who smoke less than one pack per day
- 7 mg as part of the step-down process

Nicotine patches should be applied to clean, dry, nonhairy skin on the trunk or upper arm, usually in the morning and after removing the patch used the day before. The patches employ a step-down approach to quitting. For example, if you smoke one pack per day, you would start with the 21-mg patch and gradually "step down" to a lower dose patch over an eight-week period until you are nicotine-free.

Like nicotine gum, it is important to discuss the use of patches with your doctor, especially if you have heart disease or high blood pressure, are taking medication for asthma or depression, or are using stop-smoking medications such as Zyban or Chantix.

Allergic reactions, such as itching, rash, or redness at the placement site may occur due to the adhesive or the nicotine itself. If irritation occurs, try placing the patch on another area of the skin. If the rash persists, remove the patch and talk with your doctor.

Some people have reported having vivid dreams or nightmares while using a nicotine patch. This is easily solved by either choosing a patch that is removed at night or wearing the patch for at least seventeen hours and taking it off before bed.

■ Nasal Spray

Nasal sprays such as Nicotrol are available by prescription only. They contain nicotine and are used in a way similar to how nicotine gum is used. When a nicotine craving occurs, this type of product is sprayed into the nose. Sprays are not the best choice for those with nasal or sinus problems, such as allergies or sinusitis, because the spray may exacerbate these conditions.

■ Lozenges

Nicotine lozenges such as Commit are designed to slowly dissolve in the mouth. They contain an artificial sweetener called phenylalanine (similar to Equal) and should not be used by those with phenylketonuria (PKU) or by those with sensitivity to this product. A lozenge should be moved from side to side in the mouth as it dissolves to prevent mouth sores and should not be used within fifteen minutes of eating or drinking.

■ Medication

There is no shame in using medication to help you quit smoking. In fact, the use of Zyban or Chantix as part of a larger smoking cessation program can increase your chances of quitting successfully by up to 30 percent. These medications are available by prescription only, so talk to your doctor to see if one of these medications is the right choice for you.

Zyban (bupropion HCL) is an antidepressant similar to Wellbutrin. It was discovered to be useful as a tool to help quit smoking when patients taking Wellbutrin reported a decreased desire to smoke.

Zyban contains no nicotine. It is thought to reduce withdrawal symptoms by boosting "feel-good" chemicals in the brain and blocking some of the effects of nicotine. Most people continue to smoke for the first week while their body adjusts to the medication. The most common side effects reported are dry mouth and insomnia.

Chantix (varenicline) is a medication that blocks the nicotine receptor sites in your brain, decreasing the pleasure associated with smoking as well as reducing withdrawal symptoms. The dose is gradually increased for the first week and most people continue to smoke during this time. Common side effects of Chantix include:

- nausea/vomiting
- headache
- drowsiness
- gas
- trouble sleeping/vivid dreams

Chantix is not for everyone. It can cause serious psychological changes, such as depression, thoughts of suicide, agitation, aggression, and unusual thoughts and behaviors. If any of these side effects occur, stop taking Chantix immediately and contact your doctor.

Smoking Cessation Programs

Smoking cessation programs are available in nearly every city in the country. They are sponsored by a wide variety of organizations, such as hospitals, churches, and community organizations. Many employers also offer these programs. Most cost very little or are free, and they typically consist of a series of structured classes that provide education as well as support. When used with the other tools discussed in this chapter, these programs can increase your chances of staying smoke-free.

Smoking Cessation Support Groups

Support groups are widely available and typically do not have the formal structure of a smoking cessation program. Rather, similar to other support groups such as AA, they involve regular meetings of people who have made the decision to quit and are going through similar experiences.

What to Expect When You Quit

It takes only seventy-two hours for your body to become nicotine-free. If you are not using nicotine replacement therapy, your blood pressure and pulse will probably drop to normal levels. The oxygen levels in your blood will increase, and within just twenty-four hours your chance of a heart attack decreases significantly. Your ability to smell and taste may be enhanced and your bronchial tubes will relax, making breathing easier.

In two to three months, your circulation is improved, walking becomes easier, and your lung function may be improved. By the end of nine months, coughing, sinus congestion, fatigue, and shortness of breath decrease, as does your risk for lung infection. You may find your energy levels increased, and you may be able to do things you have not been able to do in years.

By the end of one year, your risk for heart disease is cut in half. At five years your risk for lung cancer is decreased significantly, and in ten years it is reduced to that of a nonsmoker, as precancerous cells are replaced with healthy ones.

Your Plan to Quit

Your plan to quit should be very personal and based on what will work best for you. There are, however, some methods that will increase your chance of quitting successfully.

Set a Date

Once you are prepared, set a date to quit. Make sure it is a day in which you anticipate little stress and that isn't going to put you in a social situation where you might be tempted to smoke. It is not a good idea to quit on the day of your wedding or the morning of a boys' night out.

Identify Your Triggers

Triggers are a large part of your psychological addiction to nicotine. Triggers are the things you do that always include a cigarette, such as:

- finishing a meal
- drinking a cup of coffee in the morning
- drinking alcohol
- stressful situations

Identifying your triggers will help you to quit in two ways. It allows you to anticipate problems and prepare for those times when your craving for a cigarette may become intense. For example, Peggy Sue had trouble resisting a cigarette after a meal.

"It was the hardest time for me for some reason, and I have to admit I snuck a few until I decided enough was enough. Instead of sitting in my favorite chair after supper I started taking a walk around the block. Pretty soon, instead of craving a cigarette I began to crave my evening walk. I'm up to four blocks now, have lost five pounds, and haven't picked up a cigarette since."

If you have trouble resisting smoking a cigarette with that morning cup of coffee, try tea or go out for coffee in a place where you are unable to smoke. During or after a stressful situation, try deep-breathing exercises instead of lighting up.

Make a List

Take out a piece of paper, find a pen, and list the reasons you want to quit smoking. Try making them as personal and specific as possible. Instead of listing that you want to "breathe better," say you want to be able to sit through your daughter's wedding without having to sneak outside for a cigarette. Making your reasons personal and specific will help create pictures in your mind of what you desire to help keep you from lighting up.

Get Support

It is difficult to quit smoking on your own. Let your family and friends know you are serious about quitting and need their help. Check your local newspaper for support groups in your area. Keep the meeting dates and phone numbers handy. Enroll in a formal program if you need more structured support. Just know that there are people out there willing and able to help.

What to Do If You Relapse

Quitting smoking is hard work. If it weren't, there wouldn't be thousands of people who try to quit and fail every year. If you relapse, consider your past efforts as practice and learn from them. If one method does not work, try another. The main thing is not to become discouraged. Research shows that it may take several tries before you are completely smoke-free. You may want to reevaluate your reasons for quitting, identify what triggers caused you to relapse and light up, and make changes in your environment or routine to increase your chances of success the next time you quit.

What If You Cannot or Do Not Want to Quit Smoking?

Even if you choose not to quit smoking, you can minimize damage to your lungs in several ways. Changing to a brand with less tar or nicotine, taking fewer inhalations, and smoking fewer cigarettes may help reduce or delay lung damage.

CHAPTER 15

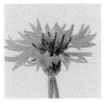

Working with the Important Members of Your Health-Care Team

By now, you probably realize you are not alone in managing the treatment of your COPD. You will form different types of relationships along your path to improved health. Some of these relationships will perhaps be new, such as with a different medical specialist or an insurance company. Others may involve a change to an existing relationship, perhaps with a friend or family member, as you invite their assistance in helping you to achieve your health goals.

The Doctor/Patient Relationship

Your relationship with your doctor or other health-care provider is no different from any other important relationship in your life. It requires open and honest communication to make it work. If you are not forthcoming about your lifestyle or your habits, it is difficult for your doctor to treat your disease effectively. Remember you are not there to impress your health-care provider, but to get treatment. Hiding the fact that you continue to smoke or are not taking your medication as prescribed only limits your doctor's ability to help you feel better.

Relationships are built on trust. You put your trust in your doctor to treat your illness as effectively as possible. In return, your doctor trusts that you will consider his or her advice, take your medications as prescribed, and be an active participant in the management of your disease. If either party breaks this trust, poor disease management will occur.

Your Responsibilities

Remember that you are an active participant in the management of your COPD. Therefore, you have certain responsibilities to those who provide you with medical care so that you receive timely and effective treatment.

Be Prepared

The days of house calls and hour-long visits with your doctor are over. Cuts in reimbursement and the advent of HMOs and PPOs require physicians to see more patients in less time if they are to remain financially viable. Prepare for your appointment ahead of time in order to get the most out of your visit. Make sure to write down any questions or concerns you have and bring them with you. It is easy to forget these things once on the exam table.

You may want to prepare a binder or folder containing pertinent information about your condition. Organizing your medical information makes it easier for you and your doctor to manage your disease. You may want to include the following information:

- a thorough and up-to-date list of your medications, including vitamins and/or other supplements and any allergies
- the names, addresses, and phone numbers of all your healthcare providers
- a complete medical history, including hospitalizations and previous surgical procedures
- copies of recent ABGs, CXR reports, EKGs, or spirometry results
- the dates of last immunizations for pneumonia and the flu
- copies of your living will or advance directive

This information is especially important when seeing a new health-care provider or specialist or when visiting the hospital or emergency room. You may want to include a blank piece of paper or bring a notebook to write down any advice or instructions they give you during your visit.

Actively Manage Your Disease
No one likes a slug. Help your doctor to help you by taking your medication as prescribed, exercising, eating healthy food, and participating in a pulmonary rehabilitation program. Be a partner in your care.

Update Your Information
Keep your records current and be sure to include your address, cell and home phone numbers, and insurance information. Pay your medical bills on time or make arrangements for payment. Most clinics and hospitals will work with you if you have financial difficulties. Remember that your doctor and his or her staff also need to eat.

Health-Care Provider Responsibilities

The doctor-patient relationship is not a one-way street. In order to provide the care and treatment regimen that works best for you, he or she has certain responsibilities to you as well.

Listens to Your Concerns
No two cases of COPD are alike. As you have learned, the diagnosis of COPD is a catch-all phrase for many forms of obstructive pulmonary disease. While your own most serious component may be chronic bronchitis, for another patient it may be emphysema. Your doctor should recognize this and treat your particular form of COPD appropriately. Only by listening to your concerns and performing the appropriate tests can your doctor provide a plan of treatment tailored to your individual needs. Your doctor should recognize that your disease is manageable and treatable and support your efforts to improve your health and your quality of life.

Orders Appropriate Tests

Your doctor should diagnose and monitor the progress of your disease as well as screen for other associated conditions by ordering the tests listed below.

■ Pulmonary Function Test

The National Lung Health Education Program (NLHEP) recommends that everyone over the age of forty-five with a smoking history be screened with simple spirometry. This test is easily performed in your doctor's office, local hospital, or respiratory testing center. Remember that the earlier COPD is diagnosed and treated the better the outcome. If a diagnosis of COPD is made, pulmonary function testing should be performed initially and then repeated every two to five years, depending on your condition, in order to track the progress of your disease and provide appropriate treatment.

■ Oximetry Test

Your oxygen saturation should be tested at rest, with activity, and at night while sleeping. Many times, a resting SPO_2 will be within normal limits but will decrease with activity. Overnight oximetry is often overlooked but should be tested so that baseline levels are documented and treated with supplemental oxygen if necessary. Studies have shown that many people with COPD have low levels of oxygen at night despite having low normal levels during daytime hours. Treating nocturnal hypoxia can increase your energy level during the day as well as decrease morning headaches and improve your mood.

■ Bone Density Screening

Bone density screening should be performed every two years, especially if you take oral steroids, such as prednisone, to manage your COPD. Steroids enhance bone loss, which can be minimized with medications such as Actonel or Boniva that help to build bone and prevent fractures of the hip and vertebrae.

■ Electrocardiogram

An EKG should be performed to search for any abnormal heart rhythms that may be contributing to your shortness of breath.

▦ Routine Screenings

Your health-care provider should help you keep up on all recommended screenings, such as mammograms and colonoscopies.

Is Informed

Your doctor should continually inform himself or herself about new medications, therapies, or procedures for those with COPD and provide you with this information as it becomes available.

Is Willing to Refer

General practitioners should be willing to refer you to a specialist when necessary. Everyone with a COPD diagnosis should see a pulmonologist. Pulmonologists are experts in respiratory disease management and can guide you and your primary-care provider, as well as keep you up-to-date on new therapies or medications as they become available. Your primary-care provider should also understand the importance of pulmonary rehabilitation and be willing to refer you for this if necessary.

Protects Your Privacy

In today's technologically advanced society, health information is easier to get than ever. Recognizing this, the Health Insurance Portability and Accountability Act (HIPPA) was introduced in 1996 to protect your private health information. Not only does this act provide standards to ensure your health information is protected but it also gives you much more control over your medical information.

The Privacy Rule protects all protected health information (PHI), including all identifiable health information gathered, stored, or transmitted by health-care organizations or providers. Identifiable information is defined as any health records that identify you as an individual with specific health problems. It does not include information contained in educational or employment records.

Health-care providers have a duty to protect this private information. They are required by law to provide you with a copy of their privacy practices. Failure to do so may result in costly fines. PHI may be used without permission only if it is a necessary part of treatment, payment, or health-care operations.

HIPPA has caused a lot of frustration for friends or family members with a loved one in the hospital. Without verbal or written permission from you, health-care providers are unable to discuss any information regarding your medical condition except in general terms, even if you are hospitalized and unable to grant permission. Before you become ill, you may want to designate, in writing, someone who will be allowed to obtain information and act as a spokesperson to other friends and family members.

What If I Am Unhappy with My Care?

If despite your best efforts you are unhappy with your physician, you have the right to find a new doctor. Research physicians in your area. The best way to find a doctor whom you will be comfortable with is by asking others with COPD for recommendations.

Medical Insurance

Could they make it any more confusing? Medicare, PPOs, HMOs, Medicaid, and private insurance companies like Blue Cross all have their own rules, regulations, and policies that seem designed to prevent care rather than encourage it. Having a general understanding of how insurance companies reimburse for care can decrease your frustration levels when dealing with these entities.

Medicare

The Medicare program was signed into law in July 1965 to provide health coverage for those on Social Security. One year later, it was expanded to include those with permanent disabilities and those with end-stage renal disease. Medicare provides partial coverage for approved medical services and contains four parts: Part A for hospital coverage, Part B for coverage for physician visits and other auxiliary services, Part C called Medicare Advantage, and Part D, which is Medicare's prescription drug plan.

■ **Medicare Part A**

Medicare Part A provides coverage for in-patient hospital services, including inpatient rehabilitation as well as medically necessary home-health services and hospice. It also covers a limited number of days in a skilled nursing facility.

You are automatically enrolled in Medicare the first day of the month that you turn 65 years of age and begin receiving Social Security benefits. If you are under age 65 and disabled, you are enrolled the first day of the month that you receive Social Security Disability benefits. If you are older than age 65 and choose to delay benefits or have not paid Medicare taxes while working, you may enroll in Medicare, but monthly premiums or co-payments may apply.

Medically necessary home-health services such as physical therapy, occupational therapy, or nursing care are covered for the first 100 visits. Hospice is covered for those with a terminal illness and a life expectancy of six months or less, and it includes a wide variety of services, including home nursing care, medical equipment, and prescription medications.

■ **Medicare Part B**

Medicare Part B provides partial coverage for medically necessary services, including:

- physician visits
- outpatient services
- diagnostic tests
- home-health services
- medical equipment such as oxygen, nebulizers, and hospital beds

As with Part A, you will be automatically enrolled in Part B the first day of the month you begin to receive Social Security benefits. If you are over age 65 and have delayed or do not receive Social Security benefits, you may enroll in Medicare Part B during the general enrollment period, which typically begins on January 1 and ends March 31 of each year. There are other special enrollment periods for those who qualify. It is important to enroll during the approved enrollment period or a life-long increase in premiums will be applied.

Medicare Part B typically covers 80 percent of approved medically necessary services and equipment and requires monthly premiums and a yearly deductable. However, neither part of Part A or B includes coverage for:

- cosmetic surgery
- medical services provided in foreign countries
- routine checkups
- hearing tests
- long-term nursing home care
- routine eye exams or eyeglasses
- immunizations

■ Medicare Part C

Also called Medicare Advantage Plans or sometimes Medi-gap, Medicare Part C is managed by private insurance companies who have been approved by Medicare. These plans include Part A and Part B coverage and may cover other services such as prescription medication. This program requires voluntary enrollment. The monthly premiums and co-payments vary from plan to plan. You can easily compare plans by visiting Medicare's website at www .medicare.gov and clicking on "Compare Plans" or by calling (800) Medicare (633-4227) and saying "agent" when prompted.

■ Medicare Part D

Medicare Part D is Medicare's Prescription Drug Plan. It is designed to help with the cost of prescription medication. The program is administered through private insurance companies so costs, co-payments and deductibles vary. If you are enrolled in Medicare Part A and have supplemental insurance through a pension or employer or are on Medicaid, you may not need to enroll. If you choose to enroll, be sure to do so during the approved enrollment period or a lifelong increase in your premiums may apply. Visit Medicare's website for a more detailed description of Medicare's Prescription

Drug Program. The website contains vital information about prescription coverage. In addition, many senior centers, hospitals, and insurance companies provide seminars that outline your options for coverage. Get help from an expert if necessary, because the plan can be confusing.

■ Medicaid

The Medicaid program was created at the same time as Medicare to provide medical coverage for those with low incomes and few resources. The program is state managed and program benefits vary from state to state. Eligibility is determined by income, and if you qualify, the program typically covers the medically necessary expenses that Medicare does not cover, such as eye exams, eyeglasses, and dental care. Check with your local department of health and human services for more information.

Friends, Family, and Significant Others

These loved ones can be your greatest ally or your worst detractor. It may seem sometimes that COPD is a disease surrounded by blame and shame. There are those who may believe you got what you deserve for smoking or that you overreact with panic when you become short of breath, which can be frustrating.

Many times, this negativity or lack of understanding comes from the same emotions you feel when dealing with your disease. Perhaps others feel guilty because they brought you that carton of cigarettes every week or angry because you continued to smoke despite their pleadings. These emotions can affect how you are treated, just as your emotions affect how you manage your disease.

While you cannot make others change how they feel, you can help them to gain a better understanding of what you are going through. Tell them how you feel or ask them to read this book to better understand your disease. If their negativity persists, you have to ask yourself if the relationship is worth the distress. You may need to let go of this person emotionally to reduce your stress and the symptoms of COPD that follow.

Luckily, there are plenty of people out there willing and able to give you the emotional support you need, if not in your immediate circle then from a wide variety of support groups such as the Better Breathers Club. This support group, sponsored by the American Lung Association, has chapters throughout the United States. Anyone affected by chronic pulmonary disease may join. The Better Breathers Club typically meets once a month and provides a forum for emotional support, education, and companionship.

Choosing a Home-Care Provider

Unless you are enrolled in a Medicare Advantage Plan, you may choose which provider best suits your needs. It may be easier to obtain all of your supplies from one provider if possible or you may get home health from one agency and decide you are unhappy and wish to make a change. Ask the following questions when making your decision to ensure you receive the type and quality of care you need:

What is their reputation in the community? This is where friends, family, or members of your support group can come in handy, as can the recommendation of your health-care provider. Ask what your supporters' experiences have been with the company you are considering. You may also check with your local Better Business Bureau to determine if the provider has had complaints filed against it.

What certifications do they hold? Several agencies accredit health-care providers. Probably the best known is The Joint Commission (previously called The Joint Commission on the Accreditation of Healthcare Organization [JCAHO]). This and other agencies are responsible for ensuring certain standards of care. Accreditation includes periodic on-site visits during which patient care and records are reviewed to determine compliance with their standards of care. Providers may hold specialized accreditations for clinical respiratory services or COPD care. Information about accreditation agencies can be found at www.medicare.gov.

Do they accept your insurance? Some Medicare Advantage Plans require you to use their "preferred provider" for home-health and medical supplies in order to receive the most complete coverage. You may choose a "non-preferred provider," but be prepared to pay a higher portion of the cost. If you are having problems with the preferred provider in your area, contact your insurance company and express your concerns. The company may allow you to switch without an increase in cost on a case-by-case basis.

Do they have certified or registered respiratory therapists on staff? Most home-health agencies do not employ respiratory therapists because there is no Medicare reimbursement for respiratory care in the home; however, some home-oxygen companies use respiratory therapists and provide their services, while absorbing the cost. If you use home-oxygen or other respiratory equipment, choose a company that utilizes the specialized skills and education that respiratory therapists provide.

Does what they offer meet your needs? If you use home oxygen and want to stay active, a nationwide provider may be your best choice because they provide seamless service when you are traveling to other cities or states.

Do they offer individualized care? An initial assessment of your needs should be performed at the first visit and addressed throughout your care. Home-oxygen companies should provide consultation regarding the oxygen system that will best meet your needs and should provide detailed instructions on the care and maintenance of your equipment.

What are their hours? They should have someone available twenty-four hours a day/seven days a week to respond to problems or concerns.

CHAPTER 16

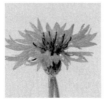

Spirituality: Finding Your Purpose, Claiming Your Power

Having COPD is difficult. The disease changes every aspect of your life—physically, mentally, and emotionally. You will need to learn how to cope with these new and often unsettling changes.

Coping with COPD

When you have COPD, you have to make many types of changes, in matters ranging from how you do your laundry to who you include in your life. Change is always a difficult thing. Studies have shown that even positive changes can cause us to feel stress, anxiety, and depression. The best way to deal with change is to accept it and find new ways to do the things you have always done. Face the changes head-on and try some of the suggestions listed below to help you through your difficult situations.

Tend to Your Spirit
Major changes in our lives, whether from disease, death, or divorce, are an opportunity for self-reflection. Often, it takes periods of adver-

sity for us to face and conquer painful emotions or gain self-esteem by meeting new challenges and rising to them. These are the times when life has slowed down and we have time for self-reflection. Be sure to do things that replenish the soul—read good books, see good movies, and build good relationships. Let go of the past and make peace with where you are in life right now. Do things that make you feel good, do things that inspire, just get out there and do…whatever it is that nourishes your soul.

Express Your Feelings

Try to build and support your important relationships with honest communication. One simple instance of miscommunication or dishonesty can lead to negative situations later on down the road. Tell your friends and family how you feel about having COPD. Ask them how they feel about it. You may be surprised to learn what they are thinking. Perhaps fear has kept them from visiting you, whereas you falsely assumed they were neglecting you because they were angry. Mend those relationships that you regret losing. You will feel better and so will the loved one from whom you have been isolated.

Laugh

Laughter really is the best medicine. Laughter can boost the immune system, improve your mood, and even help clear your lungs.

Avoid Stress

Stress kills. Stress has been linked to heart disease, cancer, and stroke. Learn healthy ways to deal with stress and keep your life as stress-free as possible. Eliminate stressful people and relationships from your life, no matter how painful. Your life depends on it.

Take Care of Yourself Physically

A healthy diet and regular exercise is necessary for your body to function at its optimal level. Eat nutritious meals and avoid caffeine, sugar, refined foods, and unhealthy fat. Eating well is essential for your body to heal and to maintain itself. Try to avoid foods containing preservatives, additives, or other unhealthy chemicals. These toxins will only add an extra burden to your immune system as it tries to eliminate them. Eat fresh fruits and vegetables, lean meat and poultry, and whole grains to keep your body healthy.

Getting regular exercise helps boost your mood as well as your immune system. Exercise releases chemicals called endorphins. These natural painkillers help improve your emotional state, cause you to sleep better, and provide an outlet for restless energy.

Take an Active Role in Your Health Care

Learn everything you can about your disease and treatment options. Knowledge can give you a sense of control over adversity. Talk openly with your health-care provider, seek information at the library, or talk with others who have been dealing with COPD. Stay on top of the latest research and new medications as they come on the market.

Accept What Is—Don't Dwell on What Isn't

Just getting out of bed can be a huge accomplishment if you are experiencing pain, fatigue, or shortness of breath. Give yourself permission to take things slow and celebrate your accomplishments no matter how small. Be flexible—it is okay to leave things unfinished. Remember that the only one you have to prove anything to is yourself. Accept that you may have bad days and you may not get much done. There will always be a good day to follow.

What Helps Others Get Through

Just as each person is affected by COPD in a different way, such as with asthma or emphysema, each person will seek different coping methods to deal with their illness. Here are stories that represent the different ways people have found to cope with their COPD symptoms.

Faith

Jean had always been very active in her church. When she learned that she had COPD, she looked to God and fellow church members for support.

"I'll admit it really shook my faith for awhile. I'd like to say that my relationship with God made it easier, but it didn't. It just seemed so unfair. Here I had worshiped God my entire life, lived by his commandments, and I felt He had let me down. I was so angry at Him for allowing me to get this disease, not to mention He wasn't giving me a cure no matter how hard I prayed. But in the end, I realized that God had not given me COPD. I got COPD because I chose to smoke. I guess at this point I should have been mad at myself, but I was so burnt out from all the anger I just couldn't work it up anymore. Luckily, my pastor and I were close. I'd been going to his church for over ten years and he asked me if I needed to talk. Thank God I took him up on it rather than going and hiding. He helped me to understand that while God couldn't provide me with a cure, He could give me the strength to deal with whatever my disease threw at me, as well as to help me find the inner peace I now enjoy."

Purpose

Marlin had never been one to volunteer; after all, he had worked over sixty hours a week for twenty years. He felt that he deserved to relax during his retirement and wanted no commitments that required punching a clock. Everything changed, however, when he learned he had COPD.

"I was diagnosed six months into my retirement. I immediately became very depressed. My wife passed away two months later and that only made things worse. I'll be honest, I did think about taking my own life. I mean, what was the point, really? I never got out of bed, let alone left the house, and my partner of twenty-seven years was gone. I guess what I wanted was to just lay there and die.

"I managed to drive everyone out of my life except for my brother-in-law Tom. No matter how surly I was he wouldn't stop coming over. We talked a lot, about my wife's childhood, the good times we shared, and how I felt about my disease. He's the one who connected me with the Better Breathers Club, a support group held at the hospital. That's when I realized that there were others out there just like me, feeling lost, alone, and depressed. It became my mission to seek them out and let them know that life can go on. It gets me out of bed every morning with a smile on my face and a purpose to do so."

Hope

When faced with a chronic illness, it can be difficult to find hope in what may seem to be a dismal future. After learning she had COPD, Norma felt like her life was over.

"We had just bought a huge motor home. It had always been my own and my husband's dream to drive all over the countryside after we retired and see as much of America as we could before we died. Learning I had COPD was a huge blow. I felt like I had ruined our plans. I totally blamed myself for getting the disease—I knew the dangers of smoking and yet I didn't quit.

"Joining the Better Breather's Club saved my life. The respiratory therapist that lives next door told me about it. It took me awhile, but I finally screwed up the courage to go. When I finally did, everyone was so nice and welcoming that I kept coming back. Meeting others who were going through a similar experience with their breathing helped me to realize that we didn't have to give up our dreams. We could still take off in our motor home and see the country. I just had to adjust my way of thinking. I made a few changes in how I did things and after that it all fell into place. We start our adventure next week and I couldn't be more excited."

Love

Love of a spouse, a friend, or a child is a powerful force. Even the love of a pet can be strong enough to motivate you to move forward in a positive way. Mary's little dog Demitri keeps her going and gives her the strength to move on in a positive way.

"Demitri is my mini schnauzer, and it may sound silly, but he is the most important thing in my life. My husband, Tom, died several years ago, and I got Demitri as a puppy shortly after Tom's death to drive away the loneliness.

"He really has been a lifesaver. I take him on daily walks so we both get our exercise, and I make sure I am on top of my symptoms because if anything ever happened to me, Demitri would be alone, and I just can't allow that to happen. He gives me a reason to get up in the morning and is always there for me when I am down. I couldn't ask for a better reason to live."

As you can see, different people have different ways of keeping their spirits up despite their COPD. Find yours and discover the inner peace and joy that you deserve.

Conclusion: In a Nutshell...

● ● ●

- Focus on what you can do rather than dwell on what you cannot.
- Feel your pain and talk about your sorrow.
- Work on managing your anger.
- Forgive yourself.
- Eat well and exercise.
- Ask for help.
- Live your life in the now.
- Cherish the good times.

Good luck and God bless.

Glossary

● ● ●

accessory breathing muscles. Muscles located in the chest, back, and shoulders that assist the diaphragm in the work of breathing.

acute respiratory failure. The point where the body can no longer eliminate carbon dioxide or provide oxygen effectively.

airway obstruction. When the bronchial tubes become partially or completely blocked due to a foreign body, allergic reaction, infection, trauma, or genetic abnormality.

allergen. Any substance that causes an allergic reaction.

alpha$_1$-antitrypsin deficiency. A genetic deficiency of the proper amount of protease and protease inhibitor resulting in a destructive form of emphysema.

alveoli. The tiny air sac at the end of the bronchioles in the lungs. The exchange of oxygen and carbon dioxide occurs here.

antibiotic. Prescription medication that is designed to kill bacterial infections.

anticholinergic. A class of medication used to relieve bronchospasm that acts upon a certain part of the body's nervous system.

antidepressant. Prescription medication that helps to adjust brain chemistry to combat depression.

benzodiazepine. Prescription medication designed to decrease anxiety.

beta-agonist (B$_2$ adrenergic). A type of bronchodilator that relaxes the smooth muscle in the bronchial tubes to ease bronchospasm.

bronchi. The two main branches leading from the trachea to the lungs.

bronchiole. One of the smaller subdivisions of the bronchi.

bronchitis. A condition in which the bronchial tubes become inflamed.

bronchodilator. A type of medication that works to relax the smooth muscle on the bronchial tubes to ease breathing.

bronchospasm. An abnormal contraction of the smooth muscle of the bronchi resulting in narrowing and obstruction.

capillaries. The smallest blood vessels in the human body. They deliver oxygenated blood from the heart to the tissues and carry carbon dioxide from the tissues into the veins.

carbon dioxide. The waste product of metabolism that is exhaled by the lungs.

cartilage. The tough elastic tissue that connects various parts of the body.

CFC (chlorofluorocarbon). Previously used as a propellant in metered-dose inhalers. Found to be harmful to the ozone.

chronic. A process that shows little change and progression over a long period of time.

cilia. Small, hairlike structures that line the bronchi. They help move mucus and small particles from the lungs.

comfort care. Medical care that focuses on making one comfortable during the final hours, weeks, or months of life.

congestive heart failure (CHF). A condition in which the heart muscle has become stressed, damaged, or scarred, making it more difficult to pump blood from your heart into your circulatory system.

cor pulmonale. Right-sided heart failure that is caused by increased pressure in the pulmonary vein.

corticosteroids. A type of medication that helps to decrease inflammation in the lungs.

diaphragm. The major muscle of breathing, it is a large band of muscle that separates the abdomen from the chest cavity. The diaphragm contracts on inspiration and relaxes on exhalation.

dry-powder inhaler (DPI). A medication delivery device that gives a dose of dry powder bronchodilator when triggered.

dyspnea. Difficult or labored breathing.

emphysema. A condition of the lungs in which air becomes trapped in the alveoli, causing them to stretch, break, and scar.

expiratory positive airway pressure (EPAP). Helps to splint floppy airways open to improve gas exchange.

exacerbation. Aggravation of symptoms or increase in the severity of a disease.

expectorants. Medication that helps to break up mucus in the lungs, making it easier to cough up and expel.

FeV_1/FVC. Ratio of FeV_1; amount of air that can be forcefully exhaled from the lungs in one second. Best indicator of early small airway disease.

forced vital capacity (FVC). Amount of air that can fully be forcefully exhaled from the lungs.

gas exchange. The exchange of oxygen and carbon dioxide in the lungs.

hemoglobin (Hgb). The oxygen-carrying protein located on red blood cells.

HFA (hydrofluoroalkane). Safe propellant used in metered-dose inhalers.

hyperinflation. A condition in the lungs when air becomes trapped due to bronchospasm or loss of tone in the alveoli, causing air to become trapped and the lungs to become overinflated.

hypoxia. Low blood-oxygen levels.

inflammation. Localized heat, redness, swelling, and pain resulting from irritation, injury, or infection.

intubation. The placement of a tube down the throat and into the lungs.

inspiratory positive airway pressure (IPAP). Assists breathing by pushing air into the lungs.

larynx. Also called the voice box; it is the entrance of the trachea.

living will (advance directive). A legal document that lets your choices regarding medical care be known when if you become unable to make them on your own. Also designates a surrogate decision maker who can enforce your decisions.

LVRS. Lung volume reduction surgery.

mast cell inhibitors. A type of medication used to relieve inflammation of the bronchial tubes.

metabolism. Biochemical processes that build the body and provide energy.

metered-dose inhaler (MDI). A medication delivery device that gives a dose of aerosolized bronchodilator medication.

methylxanthines. Prescription medication designed to relieve bronchospasm by relaxing the muscles on the bronchial tubes.

mucolytics. Medication designed to break up mucus in the lungs.

mucus. Material secreted by the lungs to trap small particles that may be inhaled.

nasopharynx. Area above the soft palate.

naturopathy. A type of therapy that stresses preventative care and uses natural methods to heal such as heat, water, light, air, massage, and often herbs and plants.

oropharynx. Area behind the soft palate and the upper part of the epiglottis.

oxygen. A naturally occurring gas that has no odor, taste, or color and makes up about 21 percent of the air we breathe. It is essential to human, animal, and plant life.

pneumonia. An inflammatory process of the lung tissue usually caused by a bacteria or virus.

protease inhibitor. A chemical produced in the lungs that deactivates, or "turns off," the effects of protease.

protease. Enzyme produced in the lungs that attacks and eats foreign matter or lung tissue.

pulmonary. Means related to the lungs.

spirometry. A test that measures the air capacity of the lungs.

sputum. Mucus and other matter brought up from the lungs.

trachea. A tube that extends from the throat to the bronchial tubes.

Bibliography

• • •

Cherniack, Reuben, M. *Management of Chronic Respiratory Disease.* Denver, CO: National Jewish Center for Immunology and Respiratory Medicine, 1987.

Daniels, Stephen. "Omega-3 Fatty Acids Can Improve COPD Symptoms." *Chest* 128, no. 6 (15 December 2005): 3817–27.

Giske, Tove, and Barbara Artinian. "Patterns of 'Balancing Between Hope and Despair' in the Diagnostic Phase: A Grounded Theory Study of Patients on a Gastroenterology Ward." *The Authors, Journal Compilation Blackwell Publishing Ltd.* (2007): 22–31.

Hodder, Rick, and Susan Lighthouse. *Every Breath I Take: A Guide to Living with COPD.* Toronto: Stoddart Publishing Co., 2001.

Hodgkin, John E., ed. *Chronic Obstructive Pulmonary Disease: Current Concepts in Diagnosis and Comprehensive Care.* Park Ridge, IL: American College of Chest Physicians, 1979.

Hsu, Clarissa, William R. Phillips, Karen J. Sherman, Rene Hawkes, and Daniel C. Cherkin. "Healing in Primary Care: A Vision Shared by Patients, Physicians, Nurses, and Clinical Staff." *Annuals of Family Medicine* 6, no. 4 (2008): 307–14.

Mullarkey, Colleen. "Alpha-$_1$ Testing and Treatment." *Advance for Managers of Respiratory Care* 17, no. 9 (November 2008): 16.

Maurer, J., V. Rebbapragada, S. Borson, R. Goldstein, M. E. Kunik, A. M Yohannes, and N. A. Hanania. "ACCP Workshop Panel on Anxiety and Depression in COPD." *Chest* 134, no. 4 suppl (October 2008): 43S–56S.

Osman, L. M., D. J. Godden, J. A. R. Friend, J. S. Legge, and J. G. Douglas. "Quality of Life and Hospital Re-Admission in Patients with Chronic Obstructive Pulmonary Disease." *Thorax* 52 (1997): 67–71.

Petty, Thomas. "A New National Strategy for COPD. Do Your Patients at Risk Know Their Lung Numbers?" *Journal of Respiratory Disease* 18, no. 4 (1997): 365–69.

Pomerleau, Cynthia S. *Life After Cigarettes*. Alameda, CA: Hunter House Publishers, 2009.

Rausch, Christopher. "Change Your Attitude, Change Your Life." *The Undersea Journal* 4th quarter (2008): 80–83.

Rossi, Andrea. "Noninvasive Ventilation Has Not Been Shown to Be Ineffective in Stable COPD." *American Journal of Respiratory Critical Care Medicine* 161 (2002): 668–89.

Spero, David. *The Art of Getting Well*. Alameda, CA: Hunter House Publishers, 2002.

Stapleton, Renee D., and J. Randall Curtis. "End of Life Considerations in Older Patients with Lung Disease." *Clinical Chest Medicine* 28, no. 4 (2007): 801–vii.

Thomas, Jay R., and Charles F. von Gunten. "Management of Dyspnea." *The Journal of Supportive Oncology* 1, no. 1 (May/June 2003): 23–24.

Wernick, Mark. "FDA Committee Recommends Pulling Primatene Mist. Does Primatene Mist Do Patients More Harm than Good?" 24 January 2006. http://www.abcnews.go.com/Health/story?id=1533708&CMP=OTC-RSSFeeds0312 (accessed 10 March 2008).

Resources

● ● ●

Alpha-₁ Foundation
2937 SW 27th Ave., Ste. 302
Miami FL 33133
(888) 825-7421
Website: www.alphaone.org
Highlights the disease and provides valuable information regarding diagnosis and treatment of this genetic form of emphysema.

American Heart Association
7272 Greenville Ave.
Dallas TX 75231
(800) AHAUSA-1 (242-8721)
Website: www.americanheart.org
Contains extensive information about heart disease, treatment options, and medication available.

American Lung Association
1301 Pennsylvania Ave., NW, Ste. 800
Washington DC 20004
(800) LUNGUSA (586-4872)
Website: www.lungUSA.org
Features a Better Breathers Club directory by state, location and meeting places, dates, and times. Provides extensive information on COPD.

Breathin' Easy—Guide for Travelers with Pulmonary Disabilities
4848 Massive Peak Way
Antioch CA 94531-8310
(925) 891-5017
Website: www.breathineasy.com

Features a guide to help travelers who use supplementary oxygen locate providers worldwide. The site also features several articles and tips on traveling with pulmonary disease.

COPD International
131 DW Highway #627
Nashua NH 03060
Website: www.COPD-international.com
Complete information regarding all aspects of traveling with oxygen, including individual airline requirements and the make and manufacturer of all approved portable oxygen concentrators.

Global Initiative for Chronic Obstructive Lung Disease (GOLD)
Website: www.goldcopd.com
Contains a valuable patient guide and questionnaire.

Medicare
Centers for Medicare & Medicaid Services
7500 Security Blvd.
Baltimore MD 21244-1850
(800) MEDICARE (633-4227)
Website: www.medicare.gov
This official government site contains extensive information regarding the Medicare program, including the prescription drug plan, eligibility requirements, billing, and more.

National Emphysema Treatment Trial
Website: www.nhlbi.nih/gov
Presents information about lung volume reduction surgery, the risks involved, and qualifying criteria.

National Jewish Medical & Research Center
1400 Jackson St.
Denver CO 80206
LUNG LINE: (800) 222-5864; Monday to Friday, 8 AM to 4:30 PM MST
Website: www.nationaljewish.org
Specializes in lung, allergic, and immune diseases. Provides information on smoking cessation, clinical trials, and much more. You

may call the LUNGLINE and speak to a nurse regarding any questions or concerns you may have.

National Lung Health Education Program
9425 MacArthur Blvd.
Irving TX 75063
(972) 920-8555
Website: www.nlhep.org
Provides information about lung function testing and spirometry, COPD, and smoking cessation.

Partnership for Prescription Assistance
(888) 4PPA-NOW (477-2669)
Website: www.pparx.org
A program that helps eligible people obtain low- to no-cost prescription medication and helps with insurance premiums and co-pays.

QuitSmoking.com
3675 Glennvale Ct.
Cumming GA 30041
(770) 346-9222
Website: www.quitsmoking.com
Features information about smoking cessation, including articles, tips, and products to help you quit. It also has a great savings calculator that calculates how much money you can save by quitting smoking.

Index

• • •

POSITIVE OPTIONS FOR CROHN'S DISEASE *by Joan Gomez, M.D.*

Crohn's disease is an inflammatory bowel condition that, while non-fatal, can be devastating. This book discusses who is at risk and why, and addresses what can be done, including self-care.

192 pages ... 1 illus. ... Paperback $13.95

POSITIVE OPTIONS FOR LIVING WITH YOUR OSTOMY
by Dr. Craig A. White

This book is a complete, supportive guide to dealing with the practical and emotional aspects of life after ostomy surgery.

144 pages ... 4 illus. ... Paperback $12.95

POSITIVE OPTIONS FOR HIATUS HERNIA *by Tom Smith, M.D.*

A hiatus hernia is a common, potentially serious condition that occurs when the upper part of the stomach pushes through the diaphragm. This book describes tests, treatments, and self-help options.

128 pages ... 4 illus. ... 2 tables ... Paperback $12.95

POSITIVE OPTIONS FOR COLORECTAL CANCER
by Carol Ann Larson

Colorectal cancer, the second leading cancer killer of adults in the U.S., is treatable if caught in time. This book tells you everything you need to know about prevention, diagnosis, and treatment.

168 pages ... 10 illus. ... Paperback $12.95

POSITIVE OPTIONS FOR REFLEX SYMPATHETIC DYSTROPHY (RSD) *by Elena Juris*

RSD, also called Complex Regional Pain Syndrome, is characterized by severe nerve pain and extreme sensitivity to touch. This book covers medical information, practical advice, and holistic therapies.

224 pages ... 2 illus. ... Paperback $14.95

POSITIVE OPTIONS FOR ANTIPHOSPHOLIPID SYNDROME (APS)
by Triona Holden

Also called Hughes syndrome and "sticky blood," APS is implicated in many serious health problems. This book identifies the symptoms and provides important information on diagnosis and treatment.

144 pages ... Paperback $12.95

POSITIVE OPTIONS FOR SEASONAL AFFECTIVE DISORDER (SAD)
by Fiona Marshall and Peter Cheevers

About 10 million Americans suffer from SAD. This book helps distinguish the condition from classic depression and chronic fatigue, and suggests ways to alleviate the symptoms and live optimally.

144 pages ... Paperback $13.95

POSITIVE OPTIONS FOR POLYCYSTIC OVARY SYNDROME (PCOS)
by Christine Craggs-Hinton and Adam Balen, M.D.

PCOS is a leading cause of infertility and affects 5–10 percent of women of childbearing age. This book covers symptoms; diagnosis and medical treatments; active self-help; and complementary therapies, including exercise, use of herbs, and lifestyle changes.

168 pages ... 17 illus. ... Paperback $12.95

POSITIVE OPTIONS FOR CHILDREN WITH ASTHMA *by O.P. Jaggi, M.D.*

This manual helps parents better understand and cope with the frightening disease of asthma, and offers advice on creating an allergen-free environment, recognizing warning signs, and the various diagnostic procedures and treatment options available.

168 pages ... 38 illus. ... Paperback $12.95

ANEMIA IN WOMEN *by Joan Gomez, M.D.*

Undiagnosed anemia in women can lead to infertility, premature delivery, fainting, and mental confusion. Joan Gomez discusses why women develop anemia more than men, the two main types of anemia, their treatment, and self-help options.

176 pages ... Paperback $12.95

THYROID PROBLEMS IN WOMEN AND CHILDREN *by Joan Gomez*

This book helps readers understand the health impact of thyroid disorders and the many treatment options. Special chapters cover pregnant women, infants and children, adolescents, and women over 50. Also discusses vitamins, the role of iodine, and the role of stress.

208 pages ... Paperback $14.95

THE IBS HEALING PLAN: NATURAL WAYS TO BEAT YOUR SYMPTOMS *by Theresa Cheung*

Information and help for those suffering from the abdominal pain, bloating, and irregular bowel habits that are the symptoms of IBS. The plan focuses on five key areas: diet, supplements, complementary therapies, stress management, and working with your doctor.

168 pages ... Paperback $14.95

SELF-HELP FOR HYPERVENTILATION SYNDROME: Recognizing and Correcting Your Breathing-Pattern Disorder *by Dinah Bradley*

Chronic hyperventilation symptoms include breathlessness, chest pain, palpitations, broken sleep, stomach problems, dizziness, and anxiety. This book explains causes and symptoms and presents a well-tested program that will help readers to breathe freely again.

128 pages ... 30 illus. ... 3rd Edition ... Paperback $13.95